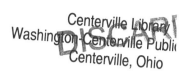

A Family Guide to Coping

with Substance Use Disorders

A Family Guide to Coping with Substance Use Disorders

DENNIS C. DALEY

ANTOINE DOUAIHY

Oxford University Press is a department of the University of Oxford. It furthers
the University's objective of excellence in research, scholarship, and education
by publishing worldwide. Oxford is a registered trade mark of Oxford University
Press in the UK and certain other countries.

Published in the United States of America by Oxford University Press
198 Madison Avenue, New York, NY 10016, United States of America.

CIP data is on file at the Library of Congress
ISBN 978–0–19–092663–2

9 8 7 6 5 4 3 2 1

Printed by Sheridan Books, Inc., United States of America

CONTENTS

This guide was written for family members, significant others, and people concerned about their relatives or friends who have an alcohol or drug problem, which in this book we refer to as "substance misuse" or "substance use disorder." We use "substance problems" to refer to drug misuse, binge (or hazardous) drinking, and substance use disorders (SUDs), a more severe form of a problem. Substance problems can take many shapes and forms and differ in their severity and impact. This family guide will help you understand these problems and how *you can help* the affected person, yourself, and other family members who may have been harmed by a loved one's substance problem.

This guide can also help individuals with a substance use problem understand the impact of their SUDs on the family as well as what their family members can do to help themselves. Addressing family issues and making amends are key issues for people in recovery from SUDs.

The first section of this guide, "Understanding Substance Use Disorders," covers SUDs from the perspective of the person with the problem. Causes, effects, treatment, relapse and recovery from SUDs, and SUDs combined with psychiatric disorders (a condition called co-occurring disorders or dual diagnosis) are discussed.

The second section of this guide, "Help for the Family Affected by a Substance Use Disorder," focuses on family issues. It looks at the effects of SUDs on the family unit and on individual members (including significant others or close friends), treatment and recovery of the family, and how to help yourself and your children if you are a parent and your children have been exposed to a parent's or sibling's SUD. We believe this guide will be a useful and effective resource for families and others concerned with a loved one's SUD. This guide can help you deal with the impact of a family member's SUD on your family unit, on yourself, and on other family members such as children. You will learn information and some practical ideas on how to cope with the challenges of having a loved one in your life with an SUD.

This manuscript could not have been completed without the help and wonderful support of Kate Scheinman and Sarah Harrington of Oxford University Press.

PART I

Understanding Substance Use Disorders

Alcohol and Drug Problems

WHO WE ARE

- *Cheryl drinks excessively on some weekends and holidays, and she occasionally smokes marijuana.* This has caused friction with her husband, Brad, who says her behavior changes when she drinks too much. Cheryl recently received a ticket for driving under the influence. Although she seldom misses work, Cheryl agrees she is not as productive after weekends in which she drinks too much.
- *Roberto, who has bipolar illness, uses cocaine regularly.* Sometimes he also drinks heavily or uses benzodiazepines not prescribed by a doctor. Roberto cut down on his cocaine use several times and even stopped a few times. However, he always returns to cocaine use even though it has led to manic behavior, depression, and suicidal thoughts. Roberto says it is hard to fight off his strong desires and cravings to get high even though he knows it is in his best interest not to use cocaine.
- *Drew got addicted to heroin after using prescription opioids for pain.* He transferred his addiction to heroin because it was cheaper. Drew uses drugs throughout the day to avoid withdrawal sickness. He engages in risky behaviors such as hustling to get money for drugs, and he shares needles. Drew has lost several jobs, and he seldom socializes with friends who do not use drugs. Drew has hepatitis C but is not receiving treatment

for it. He seldom follows through with continued treatment after completing residential rehab. He tried medications for his heroin addiction, but stopped after a few months. Drew's problem takes up much of his parents' emotional energy and time. They spent considerable money on their son's treatment, and they are perplexed as to why he won't stick with recovery. They worry that he is going to die or end up in jail. Drew's dad got so frustrated that he once told his son to get his social security number tattooed on his body so he could be identified if he overdosed and died!

- *Becky entered college with high expectations as she excelled in high school.* She was well liked by her peers and interested in a career helping others. At a recent concert, Becky trusted a friend and ingested a drug called "molly," which resulted in a fatal seizure. Her parents were devastated and confused as to why their daughter Becky, who usually had such good judgment, would try a drug like this.

Alcohol and drug problems vary in severity and how they affect different people. Cheryl's case was less severe than Drew's, yet both caused problems. Like Roberto, many people with a substance problem also have a psychiatric disorder, a condition referred to as a "co-occurring disorder." Having a substance use or psychiatric disorder raises the risk of having the other. Also, an alcohol or drug problem can worsen over time and turn into an addiction.

Even a single episode of drug use or alcohol use can lead to a severe or fatal outcome since substances affect judgment, perception, self-control, and the body's response. The case of Becky shows how a person who seldom uses drugs or drinks to excess can make one bad decision that can lead to a fatal outcome. You can imagine the heartache this senseless death caused her parents.

Many of us have family members or friends or know someone involved in a tragic outcome as a result of one poor decision from using alcohol or drugs, or from driving a vehicle while impaired. This happens far too often. Sometimes innocent victims die as a result of an automobile accident, as in the case of the young woman who tweeted "too drunk to care," and then later wrecked her car. Two friends who were passengers died in this horrible accident.

SUBSTANCE PROBLEMS

A substance problem refers to any negative outcome from prescription drug misuse, illicit (illegal) drug use, or binge drinking. These problems often lead to substance use disorders (SUDs), which involve a pattern of substance use and other symptoms or behaviors. (See Chapters 2 and 3 for these diagnosable disorders and symptoms.)

Medical or dental, psychological (mental, emotional, cognitive), family, interpersonal, social, academic, occupational, legal, financial, or spiritual problems can be caused or worsened by substance use. Any substance use can cause problems—for example, a single episode of excessive drinking or drug use can lead to a serious argument with a spouse, an injury from a fall, or even death as a result of a car crash.

WHAT SUBSTANCES DO PEOPLE USE?

People may use ANY substance that affects how they feel. This includes alcohol, tobacco products, over-the-counter medicines, and prescription medications with addiction potential such as opioids used for pain, sedatives (also called tranquilizers) used for anxiety or sleep problems, and stimulants used for attention-deficit/hyperactivity disorder. Illicit street drugs like heroin, fentanyl, cocaine, methamphetamine, marijuana, spice or K2, molly, bath salts, LSD, and many other drugs are also used.

People who use drugs often use more than one substance, which is called polysubstance use. For instance, many people who use marijuana also use alcohol, cocaine, opioids, and other drugs—even prescription drugs. The consequences of using multiple substances are hard to predict.

In addition to alcohol and tobacco, which are the most common substances used by adolescents and adults, the National Institute on Drug Abuse (NIDA) includes 25 drugs or categories on its chart of commonly abused drugs. These include drugs you may not have heard of, such as *ayahuasca* (a hallucinogenic tea made from a plant), ketamine (an anesthetic used by veterinarians that causes hallucinations), and *kratom*. *Kratom* is made from the leaves of Southeast Asian trees; the leaves are known to contain alkaloids that interact with the body's opiate receptors in a similar fashion to endorphins and opium. However, *kratom* is not an opioid but it has an opioid-like effects and can put the user at risk for opiate-related illnesses such as dependence leading to withdrawal after they stop using it.

Methods of Using Drugs

Drugs may be may be swallowed, smoked, snorted, or injected with a needle. Some people use mainly one drug while other people use multiple drugs, including alcohol. Others mix drugs together or take anything or everything to get high.

Each drug has potential short- and long-term effects, which impact the behaviors of the drug user. Some drugs have been studied, while others we know little about. Even if the public is fully informed about the dangers of a specific drug such as fentanyl (called "heroin on steroids"), people who use drugs, especially those with an SUD, will continue to use the drug for the intense high that it provides.

For information about drugs, go to www.drugabuse.gov and click on "Drugs of Abuse." This section of the NIDA website provides summaries of each drug classification, information about the effects of each drug, and current research.

WHY DO PEOPLE USE DRUGS OR ALCOHOL?

Many people who drink are able to limit their alcohol use and enjoy it without having any problems from drinking. Some people even use illicit drugs like marijuana and do not show a problem or become addicted.

People with substance problems use alcohol or drugs for many reasons, including getting high; feeling euphoric; changing perceptions; fitting in with others; and self-medicating for anxiety, depression, or sleep difficulties. In cases of physical addiction, people may use to avoid getting sick with withdrawal symptoms. Individuals with severe opioid or other substance addictions will engage in risky and illegal behaviors to get drugs and avoid withdrawal ("dope sickness"). They may lie, cheat, deceive, sell drugs for money, exchange sex for money or drugs, steal medications from family or friends, steal from others and sell these items, or rob people or businesses. Once people become addicted, their alcohol or drug use defies logic. They use for any and all reasons. For many, stopping drug use is unbearable or extremely difficult. Being without drugs can feel worse than the negative effects of the drugs.

Some users exaggerate or lie about their symptoms to doctors in emergency rooms, hospitals, or clinics. Medical professionals addicted to drugs may even steal these from patients who have been prescribed medicine for pain or other medical conditions.

The real issues are a person's reasons for using, and whether her substance use is part of a substance use disorder. As family members, we often think about the drug as being the problem when it is really the person's pattern of use and reasons for using that are the problems. Drugs come and go and are replaced by new ones all the time. SUDs and addiction are "people" problems that involve drugs.

Drug Misuse

Drug misuse refers to using other people's prescription drugs, using more drugs than prescribed, using illicit drugs, mixing drugs, or using drugs with alcohol that when taken together raises the risk of a negative outcome. As we will show in a later section of this chapter there are high rates of misuse of prescription and illicit street drugs in the United States. However, not all misuse leads to an SUD.

Addiction

Addiction is a more severe form of an SUD that involves a number of symptoms (discussed in Chapter 3). This usually (but not always) involves physical addiction to one or more drugs. For some people with an addiction, their daily lives are dominated by activities related to getting, using, and/or recovering from the effects of the drugs they use. However, addiction manifests in many different ways even though people may have similar symptoms. It may be obvious with one person, yet hidden in another person. There is simply no one way to describe addiction. Professional organizations such as the American Society on Addiction Medicine (ASAM) and NIDA define addiction as a brain disease that involves compulsive substance use leading to negative outcomes.

PRESCRIPTION AND ILLICIT DRUG USE

We are a drug-using society in many ways. According to a recent study by the Substance Abuse and Mental Health Services Administration (SAMHSA), there are high rates of use of four medications with addiction potential: opioids, sedatives, anxiolytics, and stimulants. Over 119 million adults in the United States used these drugs in 2015, over 20 million misused them, and 8% to 12% became addicted. The average North American has about a 15% chance of developing an addiction in the course of her lifetime. While the majority of people prescribed these medications do not misuse them or become addicted, many do misuse these or become addicted.

The use of opioid prescriptions has decreased since 2013, but the rates of use are still high in the United States. Many people who use these drugs do not get them from a physician for a medical condition; rather, they obtain these drugs from family members, friends, or drug dealers. As we explain in Chapter 3, a drug user's decisions play a role in whether a problem with opioids develops. Even though some people blame others for their drug problem, these users made the initial decision to use illicit or prescription drugs with addiction potential. For example, if a dental professional writes a 14- or 30-day prescription for an opioid drug following a tooth removal, the person still has to decide how long to take this medication. Some people become physically addicted due to taking opioids for pain following surgery. Everyone taking an opioid medication should become aware of both the potential benefits and the risks, especially of long-term use or use of high dosages.

Some drug users transfer their addiction from prescription opioids to cheaper, illicit street drugs like heroin or fentanyl. Heroin is distributed as a white or brown powder or as a black, tacky substance known as "black tar" heroin. Fentanyl, is potent drug that comes in many forms and is made illegally in labs throughout the world, is a synthetic opioid that is similar to morphine. Unlike heroin, fentanyl has some accepted medicinal uses as a pain medication and with other medications for anesthesia. Fentanyl is cheaper and easier to get than heroin and is often used as a cutting agent. These drugs are purchased from drug dealers or on "dark web" internet sites that sell illicit drugs and deliver them to the user's home. Rates of heroin and fentanyl use are increasing as nearly a million people now use these drugs, a rate that has doubled in the past several years. Users of these potent illicit street drugs are more likely to become addicted than those who use prescription opioids.

Users of prescription opioids often combine these with benzodiazepines, which raises the risk of overdose or negative outcomes. Alcohol, marijuana, cocaine, and other drugs are also used by those with opioid problems.

Recently, the potent drug carfentanil—a sedative used for large animals like elephants—has found its way to the streets and is often mixed with heroin or cocaine. This is a much more potent drug than all of the other opioid drugs; even a small amount can cause death.

The misuse of drugs and addiction have contributed to a significant increase in emergency room visits, admissions to medical hospitals, and admissions to addiction rehabilitation centers. In the past several years, there has been a substantial increase in the number of deaths from drug overdoses, with more people dying from this than from car accidents. It is estimated that in 2017, over 72,000 people died from drug overdoses, many of which involved prescription opioids, heroin, fentanyl, carfentanil, benzodiazepines, or a combination of drugs. Also, nearly 500,000 people die each year from nicotine addiction, and nearly 90,000 die from alcohol-related problems. Loss of a loved one often creates an emotional and financial burden for the family.

Opioid misuse and addiction contribute to family suffering, breakups, children being sent to foster care, and grandparents taking care of grandchildren because otherwise they may be removed by child welfare agencies. There has been a 5-fold increase in babies born with neonatal abstinence syndrome (NAS) to mothers with an opioid addiction. NAS refers to problems a baby experiences when withdrawing from addiction to opioid drugs that occurred in utero. Symptoms may include tremors, excessive crying, sleep problems, seizures, yawning, stuffy nose or sneezing, poor feeding or sucking reflex, vomiting, diarrhea, dehydration or sweating, and high temperature. In addition to withdrawal symptoms, the baby may experience premature birth.

In Chapter 2, we talk about the symptoms of SUDs. We discuss treatment options and recovery in Chapters 5 and 6. In Chapters 10 and 11, we discuss the impact of SUDs on families and children, and in Chapters 12 to 14, we review what can be done to help them.

THE OPIOID CRISIS OR EPIDEMIC

In recent years, a major opioid epidemic has plagued our country, creating havoc for people who use drugs, families, communities, the criminal justice system, and medical and social services providers who are inundated with problems caused or worsened by opioid misuse or addiction. This epidemic is a major health and safety problem facing our country today.

Prescriptions for opioid medications used mainly to treat pain conditions increased substantially from the 1990s until 2013. These drugs were pushed by pharmaceutical companies who promoted the idea that there were low rates of addiction among patients who used opioids. Some medical organizations and physicians believed that pain was another "vital sign" that needed to be assessed during medical visits and treated aggressively with opioid medicines. The results of relying too heavily on opioids and overprescribing them for pain created considerable harm as rates of misuse and addiction increased, leading to more overdose deaths, users transferring addiction to heroin, and many other problems for users, their families, and society.

There are a few key points that you should understand if your family member is taking a prescription opioid. There should be a legitimate medical reason for taking prescription opioids, and these should be monitored closely by the prescriber, the user, and others if this person is involved in recovery from an SUD. For most medical conditions requiring pain medication, short-term use of low dosages is recommended.

According to the Centers for Disease Control and Prevention (CDC), opioid medications SHOULD NOT BE the go-to medications for pain—except in the cases of cancer treatment, palliative care, and end-of-life care. Despite this warning, many people seek opioids for low back pain, migraines, neuropathic pain, osteoarthritis, fibromyalgia, and other conditions when nonaddictive medications or nonmedication treatments could help them.

Nonopioid medications that can be used (depending on the person's medical problem) include aspirin, acetaminophen, oral or topical nonsteroidal anti-inflammatory drugs (NSAIDs), beta blockers, tricyclic antidepressants (TCAs), serotonin and norepinephrine reuptake inhibitors (SNRIs), antiseizure medications, and calcium channel blockers.

Nonmedication treatments for pain and other chronic conditions that involve pain include cognitive-behavioral therapy; exercise; relaxation; biofeedback; physical therapy; and low-impact aerobic exercises like swimming, bicycling, and brisk walking.

If your family member becomes addicted to prescription opioids or illicit street drugs like heroin or fentanyl, treatment can help him stop his drug use, reduce his desires or cravings for these drugs, and help him learn to manage his addiction.

As we stated earlier, use of illicit drugs like heroin and fentanyl is increasing, which has led to more cases of addiction, overdoses, deaths from overdoses, and other negative outcomes. These are dangerous drugs for the user.

If your family member has an SUD, pay more attention to her behavior than to what she says. She may tell you she is not using drugs, or is involved in recovery, but she may be saying this to keep you off her back. If you notice signs of drug use, take these seriously. Talk with your family member and try to persuade her to get professional help. If she is physically addicted to an opioid drug, she likely needs supervised detoxification (also called withdrawal management) in a medical hospital, rehabilitation program, or outpatient detoxification program. However, detoxification has limited value if your loved one does not continue treatment once physically weaned off addictive substances like opioids.

OTHER TRENDS IN SUBSTANCE USE

A recent report published by the US government found that in the most recent month, 89.4% of people in the United States ages 12 or over did not use an illicit drug (street drugs or other people's prescriptions). While nearly 11% of those ages 12 or older used illicit drugs in the most recent month, 25% of young people ages 18 to 25 used these drugs, making these young people a high-risk group.

Alcohol Use

There are over 136 million current alcohol users, which includes over 65 million who binge drink (for men, binge drinking means 5 or more drinks on one drinking occasion; for women, it means 4 or more drinks on one occasion), and over 16 million heavy drinkers, who have multiple episodes of binge drinking. Over half of young people between the ages of 12 and 20 who use alcohol binge drink, and about 15% of this group drink heavily. Do not assume that it is safe to drink fewer than 4 or 5 drinks, as many people, especially those with a low tolerance for alcohol, can become intoxicated or impaired on lesser amounts. The more a person drinks, the higher his blood alcohol level (BAL) rises. As BAL rises, he becomes more impaired, and the risk of negative outcomes increases.

Marijuana Use

Cannabis, also known as marijuana is the most widely misused illicit drug in the United States and is used by 24% of all drug users. Over 115 million people have tried it, too many use it daily, and nearly 10% get addicted. Over 40% of young people between the ages of 12 and 20 have used marijuana. The majority of people with an addiction to marijuana have other substance problems as well. Also, those who develop a marijuana problem are at increased risk for developing an opioid problem. This is why families need to take seriously the use of marijuana by adolescents. Marijuana can also affect the adolescent's brain, which is still developing. This is not the safe, benign drug many people believe it is. For some people, including adolescents and young adults, marijuana can cause serious problems or increase the risk of negative outcomes such as accidents, school or work problems, family conflict, or use of other illicit drugs.

Most states in the United States have approved the use of medical marijuana, even though there is no scientific proof that this is an appropriate drug to use for many of the conditions it is approved for. Nine states have approved nonmedical use of marijuana. Many of these states show higher rates of problems with this drug since legalizing it. It poses risks for many users, especially adolescents and young people.

SUBSTANCE USE DISORDERS

Nearly 8% of the US population, or over 20 million people ages 12 or older, had an SUD in 2016. This includes 15.1 million with an alcohol use disorder and 7.4 million with a drug use disorder. Nearly 3 million people have both an alcohol use and a drug use disorder. The most common drug use disorders involve marijuana (4 million), prescription opioids (1.8 million), cocaine or methamphetamine (1.6 million), heroin

(0.6 million), and prescription stimulants (0.5 million). Community surveys show the rate of "lifetime" SUDs (meaning that people have a problem at some point in their lives, but not throughout their lives) to be much higher, close to 20%.

Treatment of SUDs

Most existing treatment focuses on the first few weeks or months, which is considered the acute phase of care. While mental health services often provide long-term treatment for chronic psychiatric conditions, many SUDs treatment programs do not provide long-term clinical services. Many people with addictions could benefit from long-term professional treatment to help sustain their recovery and manage the daily challenges they face. Short-term detoxification and rehabs help only to the extent that the person stays in treatment and/or recovery for a much longer time following detoxification or rehab.

Low Rates of Treatment Entry

In the recent SAMHSA study, only 10.6% of individuals with an SUD received treatment in an addiction specialty program that employs professionals certified to treat these disorders. While some people received medication-assisted treatment with buprenorphine for opioid use disorders in medical clinics, fewer get help for an SUD than do for a medical condition like diabetes or a psychiatric disorder such as depressive illness. Unfortunately, the SAMHSA study found that only a small percentage of people with an alcohol or drug problem believed that they needed help.

Co-occurring Psychiatric Disorders

If a person has an SUD, there is a good chance that he will also have a psychiatric disorder because there are high rates of coexisting psychiatric disorders among individuals with an SUD. Nearly two-thirds of people with borderline personality disorders, over 60% of people with bipolar illness, and nearly half of people with schizophrenia have a coexisting SUD, making these combinations of clinical conditions quite common. Also, many people with depression, anxiety, post-traumatic stress disorder, attention-deficit/hyperactivity disorder, or an eating disorder have an SUD.

SURVIVAL TOOLS FOR FAMILIES

By reading this book you should become more aware and knowledgeable about alcohol and drug problems. The more you learn, the better decisions you can make regarding how you cope with a loved one who has an SUD and your own reactions. You may learn some skills to help you deal with the challenges you face when a family member has an SUD.

We advise you to treat any episode of substance misuse or intoxication as a problem with potential negative outcomes, including the development of an SUD. Be aware of the risks associated with any episode of drug misuse, use of illicit drugs including marijuana, or an episode of excessive drinking or intoxication. Keep in mind that before becoming addicted, many people start with periods of drug misuse or excessive drinking. Too often, we passively accept a loved one's excessive drinking, intoxication, or use of drugs like marijuana because we don't think they are that harmful.

For any concerns you have about a loved one's alcohol or drug use, talk with a trusted relative, friend, other family member in recovery, or a professional to get another person's perspective. Engage your loved one in a conversation about your concerns in an empathic, nonconfrontational, respectful, calm, and compassionate manner because your relative may need your help whether she realizes it or not. You are likely to push your family member away if you threaten or attack her in a hostile manner or show poor self-control.

If your family member listens to you and changes his substance use, or gets help if a more serious problem exists, this is the beginning of the recovery process. If your loved one ignores you, this does not mean he won't make a change later. You just don't know if or when a change will be made, so you are likely to feel worried and frustrated. Furthermore, you need to stay vigilant and identify any windows of opportunity to encourage your loved one to seek help. You can also get support for yourself from others who have experienced SUDs in their families. These other people can be relatives; friends; or members of mutual support programs for families such as Al-Anon, Nar-Anon, and others. Members of family programs can provide you with education, support, and help during times of crisis. In addition, Al-Anon and Nar-Anon offer a 12-step program of change that helps you focus on yourself and managing your own reactions to your loved one's SUD. You can also get help from a therapist or counselor who understands SUDs and how to help struggling families.

Avoid labeling your loved one with the SUD as an "addict," "abuser," "alcoholic," and so on. Labels are harmful and do not matter. They stigmatize people. The same is true for the black-and-white approach to the substance problems. Searching for "magic bullets" is not the right approach. We strongly encourage you to be open-minded and hopeful while reading this book. SUDs are highly treatable conditions, and a majority of people who struggle with SUDs recover and change many aspects of their lives, including family and social functioning.

2

Substance-Related Disorders

SUBSTANCE-INDUCED DISORDERS

Substance-induced disorders include intoxication, withdrawal, and other substance- or medication-induced mental disorders such as depression, anxiety, or psychotic symptoms that are associated with use of specific types of substances. When the substances are stopped, the symptoms get better or go away altogether. A person with these symptoms could at first appear to have schizophrenia, mania, or depression when in fact the symptoms are caused by the effects of the drugs. For example, Franklin was taken to the psychiatric emergency department after becoming psychotic and stating that people were trying to kill him. He couldn't focus his attention on having a normal conversation and often talked in ways that made no sense. His friend who took him to the emergency room told the medical staff that Franklin had been using the synthetic drug called spice or K2, which often caused bad reactions such as the one Franklin was having now. Once his system was clear of this drug, Franklin no longer exhibited psychotic symptoms.

Intoxication

Intoxication shows in physical symptoms that impair judgment, affect, and mood, and it influences behavior and self-control. For example, someone with alcohol intoxication may have slurred speech, poor coordination, unsteady gait, poor memory, mood swings, or inappropriate behaviors. While our society accepts alcohol intoxication more readily than drug intoxication, alcohol intoxication can lead to many bad outcomes, even from a single episode of drinking too much.

Withdrawal

Physical withdrawal from dependence on substances can occur when the amount of use is reduced or stopped. Symptoms depend on which substances a person is addicted to. For example, withdrawal from alcohol or sedatives such as benzodiazepines can be dangerous or life-threatening due to the possibility of seizures or convulsions. Withdrawal from heroin or prescription opioids is not as risky but is extremely uncomfortable and painful: Sometimes withdrawal from opioids can lead to severe dehydration and serious health consequences. The person withdrawing may feel a strong compulsion to use to relieve the suffering, which makes it hard to get off and stay off the drug. This "dope sickness" may lead the person to do many things to get drugs to stop or avoid withdrawal. This is why detoxification from alcohol, sedatives, or opioids is needed.

SYMPTOMS OF SUDs

SUDs include disorders related to the use of alcohol, caffeine, cannabis, hallucinogens, inhalants, opioids, sedatives, hypnotics or anxiolytics, stimulants, tobacco, and other (or unknown) substances. An SUD refers to having a pattern of alcohol or drug use with at least 2 of these 11 criteria:

1. *Uses more alcohol or drugs than intended (also called "loss of control"). Examples*: John stops after work to have a few beers but cannot stop until he consumes many more. Amber was prescribed opioid pain medications for 2 weeks but continued to take them for months and became physically addicted.

2. *Has a persistent desire to quit, but has not been successful in cutting down or stopping alcohol or drug use. Examples*: Daryll stopped smoking marijuana at least four times, sometimes for several months, but he always returns to using. Melissa really wants to reduce or quit drinking, but she can't seem to reduce how much she drinks or stop for more than a few days at a time.

3. *Spends a great deal of time getting, using, or recovering from the effects of alcohol or drugs. Examples*: Adrienne spends most of her day hustling to get money to pay for heroin, getting high, or figuring out how to get her next fix. Josh sometimes misses work on Mondays following weekends of heavy drinking.

4. *Experiences cravings, strong desires, or urges to use alcohol or drugs. Examples*: Even though Dan has not used cocaine for several months, he still gets intense cravings to use. Felicia describes the first several weeks of recovery from addiction to pain medications as "pure hell because I feel such a strong obsession or desire for the drug."

5. *Fails to fulfill obligations at work, school, or home due to recurrent alcohol or drug use. Examples*: Michelle, a college athlete, often skips classes late in the week to party, and she has also missed some practices due to hangovers. Brandon was fired for missing too much work, which he says was caused by his addiction to cocaine.

6. *Continues to use alcohol or drugs despite the fact that social or relationship problems are caused or worsened by this use. Examples*: Kwan, who has a severe drug problem, refused to get help when his wife begged him to do so. Even though she left him, Kwan continued to use drugs. Jennifer continues to drink large amounts of alcohol even though her fiancé is worried that she's ruining her health and their relationship.

7. *Cuts down on or stops participating in important activities (social, recreational, occupational) due to alcohol or drug use. Examples*: Mel seldom socializes with her cousins or friends who

do not get high. As David's addiction progressed, he stopped working out and playing basketball.

8. *Uses alcohol or drugs in situations where it is physically dangerous. Examples*: Kiara often drives a car when she is intoxicated. Paul uses stimulant drugs when he goes on long car trips.

9. *Continues to use alcohol or drugs despite having a medical or psychological problem likely to have been caused or worsened by such use. Examples*: Jason uses cocaine and marijuana even though these drugs interfere with his recovery from bipolar illness and have contributed to his admission to a psychiatric hospital due to suicidal thoughts and behaviors. Ellen continues weekend binge drinking even though she experiences blackouts and cannot remember much of what happened during the drinking episode.

10. *Needs more alcohol or drugs to achieve the desired effect, or experiences a diminished effect with the same amount of alcohol or drugs (tolerance). Examples*: Alicia drinks significantly more alcohol now than in the past before she feels buzzed up. Jim, who used to drink a fifth of liquor at a time, gets intoxicated on much less alcohol now.

11. *Experiences withdrawal symptoms when cutting down or stopping alcohol or drug use. Examples*: Myra gets the "shakes" when she stops drinking alcohol. She often starts the day with a few belts to calm herself in the morning. Raymundo shoots heroin regularly not only to feel euphoria, but also to prevent opioid withdrawal symptoms.

The level of severity is classified as mild (2 or 3 symptoms), moderate (4 or 5), or severe (6 or more). Moderate or severe use is often considered "addiction," which signifies a more serious problem.

Some people do not show the symptoms of physical withdrawal sickness or medical problems associated with the disease. Their problems can even be hidden.

HOW COMMON ARE SUDs?

According to a recent study by the Substance Abuse and Mental Health Services Administration (SAMHSA) of individuals 12 years or older who used alcohol or drugs in 2016, over 20 million people developed an SUD, which is a condition with specific symptoms and different levels of severity. An SUD causes problems and distress for the user and often for other people as well. (See Chapter 4 of this guide for the effects of SUDs.) The number of individuals having specific SUDs is as follows:

- 15.1 million: Alcohol use disorder
- 7.4 million: Any drug use disorder (including prescription drugs)
- 4.0 million: Marijuana use disorder
- 1.8 million: Opioid use disorder (prescription pain pills)
- 1.6 million: Cocaine or methamphetamine use disorder
- 0.6 million: Heroin use disorder (some other studies show higher rates)
- 0.5 million: Stimulant use disorder (prescription stimulants).

This report also found that only 10.6% of these people received treatment in an addiction program. While some receive treatment in a medical setting, the majority of people with an SUD never receive professional help. Unfortunately, almost everyone with an alcohol or drug problem believes they DO NOT need help.

WHAT CAN FAMILY MEMBERS AND CONCERNED SIGNIFICANT OTHERS DO?

It is not your responsibility to diagnose a loved one's SUD. However, the more you are aware of the severity of the problem, the more you can encourage and help him get treatment. If your family member has an addiction to heroin, prescription opioid medications, alcohol, or tranquilizers, he may need medical help to wean off these drugs safely through a detoxification treatment. A person with an opioid addiction may need medications like methadone, buprenorphine, or naltrexone to help stabilize his opioid addiction and move forward in recovery. More severe forms of addiction may require a residential or outpatient rehabilitation program to jumpstart recovery.

You can help your loved one arrange for an evaluation by a certified addiction professional to determine what level of care is needed. If possible, go to the appointment with your relative to share your perspective on the problem as well as to provide support.

Depending on how motivated they are to change, people use different approaches to address their substance problems. Most people struggle with ambivalence about making change—and this is normal. If your loved one refuses your efforts to help, a professional can help you figure out strategies to encourage your relative to get help and can also help you deal with your reactions to the problem and suggest ways to cope with a difficult situation. The assumption that people can't be helped until they "hit bottom" is simply mistaken. Interventions by family members, brief counseling, and advice can make a difference in mobilizing "unmotivated" individuals. We cannot afford to wait for the person suffering as a result of drug problems to get motivated for change. Strategies to help families engage a loved one in treatment are discussed in Chapter 7.

Some communities and organizations have volunteers who are trained to provide support and help to you and your family. This may include educational and support groups for families in which members of multiple families meet with a professional to learn about SUDs, how to help your loved one with an SUD, and how to help yourself or other family members who are upset due to the substance problem. Or such assistance may include a meeting or phone call to help families discuss strategies to help their loved ones with SUDs or to help themselves. See the Appendix at the end of this guide for resources that can help families.

3

Causes of Substance Use Disorders

WHO WE ARE

- *Jordan started drinking at age 13, started using pot at 14, and became addicted to cocaine at 19.* In his 20s he got addicted to pain pills, then transferred his addiction to heroin. Jordan and both of his brothers became addicted. Their father died from medical complications related to a lifelong alcohol problem. Addiction hit this family hard.
- *Nicole increased her drinking in her early 30s and developed an alcohol use disorder.* Her drinking caused problems at home and at work, and it harmed her health. Nicole tried to quit on her own several times, but just couldn't stop. Her parents were perplexed because no one else in the family misused alcohol or drugs.
- *Logan took medications for anxiety for many years.* He got prescriptions from several doctors and never told them the truth about how much medication he was using. Logan also filled his prescriptions at different pharmacies. He did not get help until his primary care physician figured out that Logan was using greater quantities of these prescription drugs than he initially admitted.
- *Sofia started using stimulant pills in college when a friend gave her some to stay up and cram for final exams.* Over the next several

years, Sofia became addicted to prescription stimulants, and then later got addicted to methamphetamine, which almost ruined her life until she got professional help and engaged in recovery.

- *After retiring from teaching, Jodi increased the amount of wine she drank before dinner, consuming enough to feel mildly intoxicated.* Although she did not drink large amounts, Jodi's alcohol use caused friction with her husband and adult children.

These examples show that SUDs take many forms, and there are many reasons why an individual develops a problem. Substance problems can begin at any time in life. Some people, like Jordan, develop a problem early in life and come from families in which rates of addiction are high. Senior citizens like Jodi may drink more after they retire and eventually develop an alcohol use disorder. Others, like Logan or Sofia, start using drugs with addictive potential prescribed by a doctor, or given to them by a friend or relative. Over time, they develop an SUD, even to the point of physical addiction. These examples also show that the severity of an SUD varies. For some people, it dominates their lives, causing significant health and family problems. For others, it causes less damage yet the potential is there for a problem to worsen.

Having an SUD is not a matter of weakness, lack of willpower, or being "bad." SUDs result from a complex interaction of biological genetic, psychological, social, and cultural factors. These disorders are common in some families, so scientists believe a person inherits a predisposition or vulnerability to SUDs that interacts with environmental factors, which increases the risk of developing a problem.

FACTORS INFLUENCING THE DEVELOPMENT OF SUDs

Neurobiological or Physical Factors

Addiction, a more severe form of a SUD, is considered to be a "brain disease" that disrupts the part of the brain responsible for experiencing normal pleasure, controlling thinking, solving problems, managing emotions, and relating to others. Frequent use of drugs may cause changes or dysfunction in brain circuitry and stress systems, levels of brain neurochemicals such as dopamine and opioid peptides (also called neurotransmitters), and the stress-response system. Repeated use of a substance can affect major structures in the brain such as the prefrontal cortex, which is our higher-order region that is responsible for decision making (executive functions) as well as personality characteristics that emerge from that part of the brain. Adolescent and young adult brains are more vulnerable to drug use than adult brains and are less able to control behaviors.

Alcohol and other drugs create a disruption in the brain's reward system (limbic system) and provide positive reinforcement from the substance(s), which can lead to continued use despite problems. Substance use may become more important than natural rewards from eating, sex, socializing, positive experiences, or accomplishments. This is why a person addicted to illicit opioids like heroin or fentanyl will use drugs regardless of the risk of a fatal overdose.

A person's body may react differently to the way substances are metabolized or processed in the body. For example, for a person like Nicole who has an alcohol addiction, the result of her drinking may lead to an inability to respond to body cues that too much alcohol has been consumed. Genetic and environmental factors can make the brain circuitry and stress systems more vulnerable to developing an alcohol addiction.

SUDs may result from the use of prescription pain pills, sedatives, sleeping pills, or diet pills used to treat a medical or psychiatric disorder. Prescription drug problems are common in the United States even though many people who misuse these drugs do not get them from a doctor. They get them from family or friends, or buy them on the street or internet.

Psychological Factors

Factors that impact substance use and whether a problem develops include the user's personality; attitudes and beliefs about alcohol or drugs, oneself, the world; and ways of coping with problems and stresses. Some people, for example, seek excitement and pleasure through drug use and risky behaviors like hustling to get drugs. Some like "action" or "living on the edge," which drug use or being part of a culture of addiction may provide. Behavioral and emotional problems that appear in youth may predict later substance use problems.

Family, Social, and Environmental Factors

These intersecting factors include the influence of relatives, friends, and the community; the culture and subcultures in which one participates; and opportunities for success. Like other medical and psychiatric disorders (such as diabetes, cancer, and depression), SUDs run in families, which means that first-degree relatives are at increased risk for developing a problem. This does not mean that these family members *will* develop a problem; it simply means that their risk for developing an SUD is higher than for someone who does not have a family member with this problem. The children of a parent with an SUD or bipolar disorder or hypertension are at increased risk for developing the illness themselves, but this does not mean that they are doomed to getting one of these diseases.

A parent, sibling, or other relative may be a "negative role model" for a child. Children pick up attitudes and learn behaviors based on what they observe in other family members. This is why prevention efforts must begin at an early age and target the child, family, peer group, and community. Annual studies sponsored by the National Institute of Drug Abuse (NIDA) show that a large percentage of high school seniors try illicit drugs. Peers can easily influence each other to try a drug. While many young people grow out of this early stage of drinking excessively or using drugs, some end up with an SUD.

SUDs affect people of every age, race, ethnicity, religion, gender, and occupation. In many respects, especially when the SUD is more severe (as in the case of addiction), it defies logic. Although certain groups are at a higher risk for developing an SUD than others, it is difficult to tell for any one person when the symptoms will develop, how severe they will be, and how they will affect the individual or the family. Some people develop a problem in early life, while others do so later in life. For some, an SUD develops gradually over years. For others, it happens quickly.

Do not be misled by thinking that your family member has to have most of the symptoms of an SUD to have a problem that needs to be addressed now. Many people with a severe SUD had only a few symptoms early in their use of alcohol or drugs. SUDs can be progressive, with more negative symptoms and problems adding up over time. Your loved one does not have to be a heavy or even a daily user to have an SUD. Do not look at isolated events; rather, look at the big picture—the overall pattern of substance use and problems.

Personal Reflection[1]

On my mother's side of the family, I am not aware of any grandparents, uncles, aunts, or cousins having an SUD. I was told that my dad's father had a severe alcohol use disorder but eventually quit. My father had a lifelong alcohol problem starting in his 20s, but with professional help, he quit at age 66 and did not drink for the rest of his life (he died at age 80). At least 4 of his 6 siblings also had alcohol problems. I am one of 6 children, and I believe that 4 of my siblings had SUDs.

An observation I have is that, of those of us brothers and sisters who do not have an alcohol use disorder, we do have a low tolerance to alcohol. We don't drink much nor can we handle much. I believe this is actually a blessing. For whatever reasons, alcohol did not have the same effects on some of us as it did on other siblings who developed problems. This shows that we have different levels of vulnerability to an SUD. Clearly environment plays a role as well, but biology may account for a substantial portion of risk for addiction.

[1]Dennis Daley, one of the authors of this book, has incorporated personal reflections throughout the chapters. Some of these reflections appear in boxes (such as this one), while others are incorporated into the text narrative. To highlight this material, we are using this different typeface.

4

Effects of Substance Use Disorders

WHO WE ARE

- *Wes has an alcohol problem but does not miss work.* He mainly drinks on weekends or days off. Even though he drinks excessively at times, he never seems to lose control of his behavior. However, his wife worries about his drinking and how their children view his drinking as they complain that their father is not around enough.
- *Once Chris started using cocaine and methamphetamine, his life went downhill as he got addicted quickly.* He dropped out of college and went from one job to the next because he got fired for not showing up for work or for poor performance. His parents feel that he is ruining his life. The woman he lives with also has an SUD.
- *When Malik smokes marijuana, he sometimes becomes more disorganized and paranoid.* He then refuses to take antipsychotic medications for his schizophrenia. It is only a matter of time before he ends up in a psychiatric hospital. Malik's mother feels like his recovery from schizophrenia is compromised when he smokes marijuana. Once he addressed his drug problem, Malik was able to better manage his schizophrenia.

- *Elena's heroin addiction dominated her life.* She engaged in risky anonymous sexual behaviors and sold drugs to support her addiction. Her physical and mental health deteriorated. The last time she ingested drugs, she died from an overdose of heroin and fentanyl. Her parents are heartbroken because Elena had so much potential. They tried to warn her when she got involved with a drug-using crowd, but to no avail. Her mother feels guilty and wonders if she could have helped prevent her daughter's overdose.

- *Sarah is well respected as a family physician.* Her patients thought highly of her and she worked hard to establish a successful practice. During evenings and weekends when not on call, Sarah sometimes drank excessively. This affected her moods and behaviors, and upset her husband and children. Sarah started treatment, but at first she minimized her drinking. After keeping daily drinking logs for several months, however, it became clear that Sarah could not sustain any period of moderate drinking— and often drank heavily. Her husband and children began to attend some therapy sessions with her, and everyone agreed that Sarah was more involved with her family when she didn't drink. It took time, but Sarah embraced the goal of not drinking at all, and she continued in therapy and a mutual support program.

SUBSTANCE PROBLEMS AFFECT PEOPLE DIFFERENTLY

Effects of an alcohol or drug problem vary from mild to moderate to severe, and even to fatal, in cases such as Elena, who overdosed and died. Wes was able to function, and his alcohol problem was in the mild range. As with any mild problem, however, there is a risk that it can worsen over time and lead to addiction. Chris's and Malik's problems were more severe, with numerous negative outcomes. Due to Malik's psychiatric condition, he is more vulnerable than others to have a bad outcome from using small amounts of marijuana. Sarah functioned at a high level as a physician, but her drinking was excessive and worried her family.

The effects of a substance problem on the person with the SUD or on the family depend on a combination of factors, including:

- Amount, frequency, and methods of substance use
- Presence of a co-occurring medical or psychiatric disorder
- Behavior and functioning
- Exposure to trauma
- Quality of relationships and social support
- Positive life experiences
- Access to treatment and recovery and willingness to stick with it
- Motivation for change.

Amount, Frequency, and Methods of Substance Use

Types, quantity, frequency, and methods of substance use help determine the nature and severity of the problem. Substances can affect your loved one's ability to function—his judgment, emotions, behaviors, and self-control. A daily user of large amounts of alcohol or drugs is likely to experience more problems than someone who is not a daily user or does not ingest large quantities of substances. Your family member is also likely to be a burden on the family.

> In my family,[1] my father often drank a case or more of beer over a period of a day or two, usually on the weekends (although he also drank during the week when not working). His alcohol problem was severe as it harmed his health, ability to work, and his family relationships. He often missed work or lost jobs as a result of drinking binges. My family was poor and relied on welfare from time to time to help pay the rent and supply us with surplus foods, then food stamps.

[1]Dennis Daley, one of the authors of this book, has incorporated personal reflections throughout the chapters. Some of these reflections appear in boxes (such as the one in Chapter 3), while others are incorporated into the text narrative, such as we see here. To highlight this material, we are using a different typeface.

Presence of a Co-occurring Medical or Psychiatric Disorder

Studies show high rates of co-occurring problems in individuals with SUDs. Each of the types of problems—substance use, psychiatric, or medical—can be mild, moderate, or severe. Some psychiatric disorders affect the person's decision-making ability, thoughts, emotions, and behavior. This, in turn, can contribute to bad decisions and outcomes from using drugs that make psychiatric symptoms worse. Families with members who have multiple disorders are more prone to worrying about their loved one.

My father stopped drinking after he was treated by a friend and colleague—an addiction psychiatrist—for his alcohol use disorder, a depressive disorder, and an anxiety disorder. I believe that my father probably would not have sustained his recovery if his psychiatric disorders had not been treated in an integrated manner.

Some people do well with their substance use or psychiatric disorder, but continue to smoke cigarettes. Jack, who worked hard and sustained his recovery from a severe cocaine addiction, did not stop smoking until he was diagnosed with lung cancer.

Behavior and Functioning

People with substance problems may function adequately at work or at home, and not seem to have a serious problem. Others become unpredictable, hostile, aggressive, violent, impulsive, or suicidal after using drugs or alcohol, and they put themselves and others at greater risk for a negative outcome.

> My father was a mild-mannered man with a tendency to be low-key or depressed when not drinking. He was like Dr. Jekyll and Mr. Hyde, who became mean, obnoxious, and sometimes violent when drunk. I watched him tear off his shirt, throw plates of food against the wall, and engage in other harmful behaviors when drunk. I believe his alcohol use disorder played a major role in his absence as a father figure and his failure to attend any school, athletic, or community functions that I or my siblings were involved in.

Exposure to Trauma

Being under the influence of alcohol or drugs can increase the risk of making decisions that expose people to potential or actual danger. For example, Maria got high with people she did not know very well. She woke up in a strange place with her clothing torn and the survivor of sexual assault, yet Maria could not remember what actually happened.

> I believe that my father suffered from post-traumatic stress disorder due to his experiences in World War II, where he was wounded (he was a machine gunner who fought in the Pacific). Dad's generation seldom talked about their military experiences, and we children did not learn much about what he went through until he was in his 70s. Exposure to trauma can raise the risk of developing an SUD or psychiatric disorder.

Quality of Relationships and Social Support

Beth lost several friends due to her involvement with a group of people who use cocaine. She stopped socializing with her friends who don't use drugs. Although Donald's son has a severe drug problem and refuses help, Donald is seeing a counselor for his own mental health. He also attends a support group for family members harmed by a loved one's addiction. Donald believes these are helping him deal with this very difficult situation.

Positive Life Experiences

Suzie, a member of a college basketball team, increased her use of marijuana and tested positive on a urine drug screen. An athletic trainer convinced her to stop smoking marijuana and get help before it got out of hand. Suzie used her energy to work harder at school and sports. Staying connected with other athletes who did not use drugs helped her as well. As she focused on becoming a better athlete and student, Suzie became more motivated to not use any drugs. After being in recovery from opioid addiction for nearly 2 years, Bruce started his own home repair business. He slowly grew his business and now employs several people because he has so much work. Bruce feels that not rushing into starting this business was a good decision. His wife agrees and both feel their quality of life has improved substantially since Bruce engaged in long-term recovery and put himself in a position to follow his dream of having his own business.

Access to Treatment and Recovery and Willingness to Stick with It

Those who address their substance problem before it becomes severe have a good chance to reduce the potential harms related to it. For those in need of treatment, sticking with it is a major factor in determining the outcome. Early dropout from treatment is usually not a good sign. Similarly, family members who get professional help and/or engage in a family support group have an opportunity to learn strategies to cope with their loved one's substance problem and its impact on themselves.

Motivation for Change

Motivation for change may ebb and flow in early recovery, both for the person with the SUD and the family. The best antidote for anyone who has a dip in motivation is to stick with a treatment or recovery program, even if he feels like quitting. Periods of low motivation usually change for the better. Ambivalence or "mixed feelings" is a normal part of motivation. Your loved one's motivation to stay in treatment or recovery can be enhanced by your caring reactions and by letting him know you understand that the recovery process can be very challenging. On the other hand, your loved one's motivation to change can be lowered if he is confronted by a family member.

It is never too late to get help! We, authors, have worked with people (and their loved ones) who recovered in their 50s or 60s and sustained their recovery for years. It is lifesaving and very fulfilling work.

> My father stopped drinking at age 66 and maintained sobriety until he died at age 80. His initial motivation to stop drinking was driven by my mother getting sick and dying from cancer.

There are many reasons and motivations for why people decide to stop using and maintain sobriety. Motivation for change is a very important dimension of addiction and recovery. Your family member has to find her own motivation. While she can initially start treatment or recovery to satisfy a loved one or to comply with pressure from the legal system or an employer, over time her motivation has to come from within herself for the change to be sustained.

SPECIFIC EFFECTS OF SUDs

SUDs can cause or worsen problems in any area of life. Problems occur as a result of substance use as well as from living a lifestyle in which the person does not take care of his physical, emotional, or spiritual health or relationships. Negative effects range from mild to moderate to severe to fatal. The pain and turmoil that SUDs can create for the individual or family can be significant. Table 4.1 lists examples of the effects of SUDs in various areas of functioning.

Many studies and surveys of individuals with SUDs document a range of negative effects on the person, family, and society, many of which were discussed in this chapter. In addition, our extensive clinical work with thousands of individuals with SUDs and their families has exposed us to about every negative effect of an SUD that can be experienced. On the other hand, studies and surveys show that participation in professional treatment, engagement in mutual support programs, or both lead to innumerable positive outcomes in all domains of health and functioning.

As I sometimes state in my teaching of professionals and discussions with groups of patients with addictions who are in treatment, I am humbled and impressed by how some individuals with severe addictions who have knocked on the door of death and visited the gates of hell have bounced back and engaged in a meaningful recovery. And even more impressive is how many of these individuals now help others, either in their professional work in the field of addiction treatment, as volunteer recovery coaches, or as peers in mutual support programs like Alcoholics Anonymous or Narcotics Anonymous.

Table 4.1 PROBLEMS ASSOCIATED WITH SUDs

Problem Area	Examples
Medical/health	Poor physical or visual health habits; accidents; injuries; poor nutrition; weight gain or loss; increased risk of liver, heart, kidney, or lung diseases; cancers of the mouth or pharynx; gastritis; edema; high blood pressure; sexual problems; complications with menstrual cycle, pregnancy, or childbirth; increased risk of HIV or AIDS, hepatitis, or premature death
Overdoses	The number of overdoses and deaths from overdoses is rising rapidly due to users mixing drugs, using potent street drugs like fentanyl or carfentanil, or taking a drug with another drug mixed in that they did not know about.
Withdrawal	Substance-related withdrawal symptoms are experienced when cutting down or stopping after regular and heavy use of alcohol or drugs for a prolonged period of time
Dental health	Poor dental hygiene (lack of dental checkups or care), gum disease, bad teeth or loss of teeth caused by substances, poor hygiene, or excessive use of sugary foods or drinks
Emotional/ psychological	Anxiety; panic reactions; depression; mood swings; hallucinations or other psychotic symptoms; suicidal thoughts, feelings, or behaviors; unpredictable actions; aggressiveness; violence; self-harm; feelings of shame and guilt; low self-esteem; increased risk of relapse or recurrence of a psychiatric illness due to effects of drugs or alcohol
Work/school	Poor performance; loss of jobs or dropping out of school; missing work or school; being undependable and less effective; loss of interest; ruined career; under- or unemployment; lost opportunities

Table 4.1 CONTINUED

Problem Area	Examples
Family	Lost relationships due to separation, divorce, or involvement of child welfare agencies; family distress and conflict; damaged family relationships; emotional burden on the family (anger, hurt, distrust, fear, worry, depression); poor communication
Interpersonal	Lost or damaged friendships; conflicts with others and dissatisfaction with relationships; loss of trust or respect of significant others
Recreational	Diminished interest in or loss of important hobbies, avocations, or other leisure activities
Legal	Fines; legal constraints; arrests; convictions; jail or prison time; probation or parole
Economic	Loss of income; excessive debts; loan defaults or ignoring other financial obligations; loss of security or living arrangements; inability to take care of basic needs for food or shelter; using up all financial resources; inability to manage money

The next two chapters discuss treatments for SUDs, as well as the process of recovery. You will learn that there are many treatment services and approaches that can help people with SUDs and many recovery resources that can help them reclaim themselves and recover.

5

Treatment of Substance Use Disorders

WHO WE ARE

- *A few years after retiring from working as a mechanical engineer, Anna increased her drinking to 2 or 3 glasses of wine before dinner.* This affected her behavior and ability to function, and caused concern among her adult children and grandkids. After hearing her adult son and daughter share their worries, Anna agreed to attend outpatient counseling to figure out what to do about her drinking. Anna attended 8 sessions over several months, and with the help of her counselor she decided it was in her best interest to stop drinking. Her adult children attended a few of these sessions to provide input about their mother's drinking and how it affected the family. Anna also attended an Alcoholics Anonymous (AA) meeting each week. She has sustained her sobriety for over a year and seldom has a desire to drink. Her children and grandkids feel she is doing much better since she stopped drinking.
- *Jared was addicted to heroin, but refused to go to rehab at the suggestion of his family.* Instead, he attended an intensive outpatient program 3 days a week for 3 hours each day. He was also offered buprenorphine but didn't want to take this medication. After several months of stopping drugs, then using

again, Jared agreed to enter a residential rehab program. He was detoxified from heroin first, and offered buprenorphine again but still refused to take it. When Jared finished rehab, he continued in outpatient treatment and did well for over 6 months before he started using heroin again. After he started using again, his parents set up an evaluation for treatment again and went to the session with him. Jared agreed to outpatient detoxification and a trial of buprenorphine. The medication took the edge off his strong cravings and enabled Jared to benefit from outpatient counseling. His parents attended some sessions with him and also went to Nar-Anon while their son attended Narcotics Anonymous (NA) meetings. Jared has not used any drugs for nearly 2 years now, sees a counselor regularly (sometimes with his parents), takes buprenorphine, and attends several NA meetings each week. His parents continue to attend Nar-Anon for their own benefit.

- *La'Valle did well in recovery from recurrent major depression and cocaine addiction for over a year.* She then met a man who convinced her she could dabble in drug use without losing control. It didn't take long for La'Valle to lose control over cocaine use. She also stopped taking her antidepressant medication. This, and the effects of cocaine, led to La'Valle feeling suicidal, so she sought help in a psychiatric hospital. During a brief inpatient stay, she restarted her medications, agreed to attend an outpatient program that focused on her addiction and depression, and accepted the need for abstinence from drugs if she was to get her life back on track. La'Valle ended the relationship with the man who reintroduced her to drugs and now socializes with others who are in recovery. She has gotten closer to her children since engaging in recovery.

These examples show that there is no single treatment or approach that fits everyone. People do not respond the same way to any one particular treatment approach in any particular setting. One size clearly does not fit all. Based on our experiences, we practice with humility; we strongly believe that clients with SUDs know themselves well and should be provided with the information they need to make informed choices about their treatment. Some people need more intensive and/or extensive treatment than others. It is not unusual for a person with a more severe SUD to engage in several episodes of treatment over time before sustaining recovery. For those who are physically addicted, medical detoxification may be needed before they can benefit from other types of treatment. Without detoxification, it may be nearly impossible for some to quit because their body craves drugs or alcohol. No matter how poorly your family member is doing, never give up because you never know if or when she will decide to get help. Individuals with addictions engage in unpredictable behaviors when it comes to making a decision to get help and address their SUDs.

HOW FAMILY MEMBERS CAN SUPPORT TREATMENT

As researchers, program developers, educators, and clinicians, we have witnessed over the past 30 years that a majority of people with SUDs change, get better, transform their lives, and regain stability. In our practice, we have also experienced the positive impact on families and concerned significant others. Family members involved in treatment and/or mutual support programs often feel better and more confident about being able to deal with a loved one's SUD.

Treatment helps the person with the SUD learn about alcohol and drugs, causes and effects of SUDs, treatment options, relapse, recovery, and community resources. Treatment also helps the person accept the SUD, learn skills to manage the challenges of recovery, and develop a long-term change plan. Skills may include changing addictive thinking or behavior, limiting or ending relationships that do not support recovery, learning to handle emotions without needing drugs or alcohol, developing a healthy lifestyle, and learning to identify and manage relapse warning signs and high-risk relapse factors.

If your family member or friend gets sick when alcohol or drug use is stopped or cut down, or has medical or psychiatric problems that may be caused or worsened by the SUD, help him seek professional treatment. This may be needed to initiate recovery.

Treatment may involve a combination of professional and mutual support programs such as AA, NA (or other 12-step programs), SMART Recovery, Women for Sobriety, or other programs. Many people do well as a result of treatment. Others derive benefits but have episodes of substance use and need multiple attempts at treatment over time to manage their SUDs. This is no different than treatment for other chronic medical or psychiatric conditions that require multiple treatments over time. Some people with an SUD are able to quit using on their own without treatment, but they usually have less severe forms of an SUD. However, if your loved one has tried on her own before and it hasn't worked, we recommend that she get treatment.

Treatment is helpful only to the extent that your loved one sticks with it and uses the guidance of professionals and peers in recovery to make changes and manage the SUD. Early dropout from treatment or recovery is usually a bad sign. Unfortunately, some people with SUDs struggle with their motivation to change and experience limited benefits from treatment, regardless of types of treatment received or how many times they engage in treatment. Others resist treatment despite the severity of their SUD. Ambivalence about change is a huge part of it. Any of these negative outcomes can cause you to have feelings of helplessness, anxiety, depression, or anger. While you can continue trying to influence your family member to get help, at some point it may be best to focus on coping with your own negative feelings and accept that you can only have so much influence on your family member.

TYPES OF PROFESSIONAL TREATMENT

The person with an SUD may use any combination of treatment programs, services, or community recovery supports. Treatment includes detoxification; rehabilitation; individual, group, and family therapy; other services (case management, vocational or leisure counseling, medical evaluation); and medications. Some individuals receive services in primary care offices and other medical practices from physicians, nurse practitioners, nurses, physician assistants, and others. These services may include screening, evaluation, brief treatments, and referrals to specialty addiction care for more severe problems. Some locations provide ongoing medications for addiction to opioids, alcohol, or nicotine. (Some refer to this as "medication-assisted treatment" [MAT]; we believe medication should be considered a treatment in itself and not something that "assists" treatment.) Community recovery supports include mutual support programs such as AA or NA or others, sober housing, and recovery clubs.

Some people need several treatment episodes over time. This does not mean they failed; rather, it means that their SUD is such that long-term involvement in treatment is needed. As individuals go through different programs over time, they may reach the point where they achieve and sustain stable recovery.

Many people ask us to recommend "good" programs for the affected family member. The reality is while some programs may be better than others in terms of providing strong evidence-based practices, these are usually short term, and the work of recovery occurs to a large extent after a person completes a program. It is really the person's investment in treatment in the program and his motivation for change that determines the outcome.

Detoxification (Medical Management of Withdrawal)

Detoxification in a medical or psychiatric hospital, rehab program, or outpatient clinic helps the person safely withdraw from physical addiction to alcohol or drugs and develop a plan for continued care. Detoxification usually lasts 3 to 7 days or longer and is managed by doctors, nurse practitioners, nurses, physician assistants, and other providers. Detoxification involves taking medications to reduce symptoms of withdrawal, getting rest, and eating well. Most detoxification programs also offer education, counseling, and planning for post-detoxification treatment. Detoxification has limited benefits if the person does not follow up with ongoing treatment and/or recovery. Most detoxifications occur in residential or hospital settings—few outpatient clinics offer detoxification.

Short-Term Residential Programs (Less than 30 Days)

Short-term residential programs provide information on SUDs and recovery, teach strategies to manage the challenges of recovery, and help the individual develop a plan for continued care. Such programs are housed in residential settings or hospitals and usually last 2 to 4 weeks, although programs for adolescents may last longer. There is much focus today on the need for more rehab beds, but the reality is rehab has limited value if the person does not continue treatment. What sometimes happens is that addicted individuals feel good after several weeks of being drug free while in rehab, and they believe that they can continue recovery on their own without the help and support of professionals or peers in recovery. In time, they go back to using because they are bombarded with cues in the environment that trigger cravings.

Long-Term Residential Rehabilitation Programs (90+ Days or Months)

Long-term residential rehab programs include therapeutic communities, halfway houses, and three-quarter-way–house programs. Long-term programs help the person continue to learn ways to manage recovery challenges, get involved in vocational training or find a job, and engage in mutual support programs. These programs are housed in residential settings and last 3 to 6 months to a year or longer. Some programs for women allow them to keep their children with them while in the program. Individuals with multiple relapses who have difficulty sustaining sobriety and those who need more time in a supervised setting can benefit from these programs, especially a long-term halfway house or a therapeutic community (some programs may be both of these). However, the person should continue engaging in recovery after discharge to help sustain gains and catch early signs of relapse.

Nonresidential Rehabilitation Programs

Nonresidential rehab programs include partial hospital or intensive outpatient programs that the person attends up to 5 days per week. Such programs help the person become educated, develop recovery skills, and formulate a plan for continued recovery. These programs can be used as a stepdown program following detoxification or rehab, or they can be used for those who do not do well with outpatient treatment (which usually happens once a week or less). These programs occur in outpatient settings and last 4 to 12 weeks or more, depending on the program and source of funding.

Outpatient Counseling or Therapy

Outpatient counseling or therapy helps people with SUDs assess their problems and determine what they want to change about their substance use. The counselor or therapist can make referrals if other programs such as a residential treatment program are needed. Outpatient counseling and therapy also are used as a stepdown from detoxification, rehabilitation, or other programs. The length of time varies from a few sessions to months or longer. These services occur in outpatient treatment clinics or private practices. Some clinics offer long-term continuing care.

Medication-Assisted Treatment

Effective medications reduce or prevent withdrawal symptoms and help persons with an addiction safely detoxify. Medications involve the use of medications approved by the US Food and Drug Administration (FDA), in combination with counseling and behavioral therapies, to provide a comprehensive approach to treatment. A common myth about the use of medications for addictions is that it substitutes or replaces one drug for another. The reality is that these medications help individuals stop substance use and address cravings and stay in treatment so they can sustain recovery.

Disulfiram (Antabuse), acamprosate (Campral), and naltrexone (Revia, Vivitrol) are the most commonly used medications to treat alcohol use disorder (AUD). None of these medications provides a cure for the disorder, but they are most effective in people who work a recovery program. These medications can help reduce craving and the risk of relapse. Another promising medication not FDA-approved for AUD is topiramate (Topamax).

There are three medications used to treat opioid use disorders:

1. Methadone (Methadose, Dolophine) is an opioid full agonist (an agonist is a drug that activates opioid receptors in the brain and does not block other opioids while preventing withdrawal). This is dispensed only in specialty regulated clinics.
2. Naltrexone (Revia, Vivitrol) is a nonaddictive opioid antagonist (an antagonist causes no opioid effect and blocks the effects of other opioids) that is dispensed as a daily pill or a monthly injection.
3. Buprenorphine (Subutex without naloxone; with naloxone: Suboxone, Zubsolv, Bunavail, and generic, Subiocade, and Probuphine) is a partial opioid agonist (meaning it activates the opioid receptors in the brain, but to a much lesser degree than a full agonist, and blocks other opioids while reducing withdrawal risk). It is dispensed as a dissolving tablet, cheek film, 6-month implant under the skin, or monthly injection.

There are three FDA-approved medications to treat tobacco use disorders (smoking, chewing, or sniffing tobacco):

1. Nicotine replacement medications, including chewing gum, transdermal patch, nasal sprays, inhalers, and lozenges, help reduce nicotine withdrawal symptoms such as anger, irritability, depression, and anxiety. Some of these medications are available over the counter.
2. Bupropion (Zyban) originally approved as an antidepressant, has also been found to help people quit smoking. It is a prescription medication.
3. Varenicline (Chantix) is a nicotine partial agonist that reduces the craving for cigarettes and has been helpful in stopping smoking. It is a prescription medication.

Medications for any SUD should be used in conjunction with therapy or counseling, mutual support programs, or both. These medications can be prescribed by professionals in addiction programs or medical clinics. Only those who receive a waiver from the FDA can prescribe buprenorphine for opioid addiction.

Mutual Support Programs and Recovery Clubs

AA, NA, and other 12-step programs; Women for Sobriety; SMART Recovery; and Alcoholics Victorious are mutual support programs that aid recovery. There are other programs as well, but they are less common.

Most mutual support programs are free, and while some are available in many areas, others are less available. Programs promote fellowship and include meetings of recovering people, the 12 Steps or other programs of change, and events such as dinners, conventions, and social activities. These programs may be used for short- or long-term involvement. Some people participate for years or even decades. This participation helps them sustain recovery and provides a context in which they can offer support to newcomers or other members whom they sponsor. Research shows that active involvement in 12-step programs has a positive impact on recovery from SUDs. Active involvement means attending meetings, using a sponsor, working the steps, and using the other tools of the program.

Your family member may resist or state that these programs do not help. Keep encouraging him to stick with it. Many people who initially do not benefit later find these programs to be helpful. If your family member will not attend a mutual support program, try to help him identify other sources of support so he does not face recovery alone.

Recovery clubs offer an alcohol- and drug-free environment in which recovering people can socialize, relax, watch TV, eat, and/or participate in social activities. A variety of 12-step recovery meetings are held for SUDs or other compulsive or addictive disorders at these clubs. When Max got sober, he found himself with too much free time on his hands. He worried that boredom could lead him back to drinking. At the advice of a friend in recovery, he went a local recovery club each day where he attended meetings, sought support from others during discussions between meetings, and spent time reading recovery literature. Max also attended weekend dances and joined other people in recovery in attending outside sporting events. Max found that this connection with others in recovery and access to a safe place to socialize and attend meetings increased his confidence level in staying sober.

Some mutual support programs provide online chat rooms that allow people to connect via the web. There are also recovery apps that can aid recovery. Many people find connection to their peers in recovery to be extremely helpful in managing their SUDs.

Primary Care and Other Medical Practices

In recent years, there has been an increase in healthcare professionals based in hospitals, emergency departments, and community primary care or specialty clinics who provide some services for individuals with SUDs. You can talk with your primary care physician (PCP) or other provider, or your family member's PCP, to find out what services she may be able to provide. Some people with SUDs prefer getting treatment in a medical system rather than in an addiction system because of stigma and other reasons. What is important is that your loved one gets help.

Limitations You May Face in Finding Help for Your Loved One

Getting help for an SUD is not always easy. Some programs are hard to get in to due to waiting lists, admission criteria, or funding. Getting help for your family member may require persistence, insistence, and talking to directors or administrators of programs when you feel that the frontline staff who handle admissions are not helping you.

WHY PEOPLE GET HELP FOR AN SUD

- *Jose got help with his drug problem because he knew he was hurting his family and wanted to keep everyone together.*
- *Marion got help because she risked losing her job if she did not.*
- *Bill decided treatment was a better choice than jail, so he agreed to attend a program.*
- *Abby got help when she discovered she was pregnant and did not want to place her baby at risk.*
- *Gary joined AA and quit drinking because he knew it was ruining his marriage and his health, and he didn't want to die early from liver disease like his father had.*

These examples show that there are many reasons why people get help for an SUD. Some realize they have a problem and decide to get help on their own. Others get help due to the encouragement of a family member or medical professional, or as a result of pressure from the court system or an employer.

Even if your loved one has serious problems caused by his SUD, he may downplay the impact of the problem. Or he may agree that he has a problem but not accept help from professionals or peers in mutual support programs. He may blame the problem on something other than his SUD. Using labels like "addict" or "alcoholic" may not make him see or accept the substance problem or even agree to get treatment; in fact, it can have a damaging effect. Meeting your family member where he is and working with him is an approach you can take rather than demanding that he gets help or change his substance use.

The very unfortunate fact is that the majority of people with SUDs do not get help. While some quit on their own (usually those with less severe SUDs), many need treatment and/or help from mutual support programs. It doesn't matter why or how people get into treatment because once in treatment, they have a chance of turning their lives around and stopping substance use. Resumption of use is common following a treatment episode and should be seen as a reason to resume treatment or even intensify it.

THE IMPORTANCE OF FAMILY INVOLVEMENT

You may wonder what good it is to persuade a family member or friend to get help. After all, what good will it do if she doesn't want to be in treatment and she goes only to save a job or a marriage, or to stay out of jail? Remember, many people struggle with admitting that they have a problem or seeking help because of shame or stigma. It is a myth that nothing can be done until a person with an SUD "hits bottom" and suffers considerably. In fact, interventions involving counselors and family members or motivational counseling can enhance a person's motivation for change. And if your relative is in treatment, even involuntarily, she has an opportunity to understand and accept her SUD.

While families and concerned significant others may hear that they can do nothing or should "detach," the truth is they *can* have an impact on their loved ones with an SUD by influencing them to get treatment, engage in mutual support programs, or both. Multiple studies show that there are several types of professional interventions that families can use to influence their loved ones to get help for their SUDs. These programs go by names such as Community Reinforcement and Family Training (CRAFT), A Relational Intervention Sequence for Engagement (ARISE), multisystemic family therapy, brief strategic family therapy, network therapy, and others. These approaches work with families individually to help them figure out ways that they may influence the member with the SUD to get help. Even if such attempts to help your relative with the SUD do not work at first, these approaches can help your family focus on dealing with your own reactions to a loved one's SUD as well as your disappointment in dealing with her resistance to getting help for the SUD. Some families even form their own intervention team without a professional, sometimes with the help of a peer such as a recovery coach.

Pressure is most effective when individuals are faced with consequences should they refuse to seek help for their SUDs. For example, the possibility of losing one's job, family, or freedom can be a potent motivator.

The reaction of individuals with an SUD to family pressure, encouragement, or reinforcement varies. Many individuals appreciate the love, concern, and courage of their families to take steps to try to pressure them to get help. Sometimes this appreciation isn't shared until the person has been in recovery for a while and it sinks in what the family did to help. Others may become angry or hostile. If your loved one threatens you or other family members or is prone to violence, it is best to seek professional guidance to help you figure out how to approach him to minimize a negative outcome, or even to decide if it is safe to try to persuade him to get help.

No single approach works for all families, so you have to find what may work for you. Family members often feel good about themselves for taking action to help a loved one with an SUD. Even if their help was refused, family members often feel and function better because they took action rather than passively accepting the problem. If your family member with the SUD resists your efforts to get help, she may still get the message that you know a problem exists and that you will take steps to make sure your own life doesn't become harmed any more.

WHAT IF YOUR FAMILY MEMBER REFUSES TREATMENT?

Your efforts to influence your loved one to enter treatment may not work this time, or may take longer than you expect. Your family member may resist, minimize the seriousness of the problem, or feel strongly that she can handle the problem without help from others.

Remember, an addicted brain does not operate with logic. Rather, it tells the person that drugs are needed to feel good or to not feel bad. An addicted brain has an impaired decision-making ability, so this person may not see the same reality as you.

Be patient and don't give up! Watch for any windows of motivational opportunity to encourage your loved one to seek treatment and then get her into treatment. Keep trying because you never know when a family member will agree to get help. She may agree to get help and then abruptly change her mind, especially if steps are not taken quickly to facilitate treatment.

IS SUD TREATMENT EFFECTIVE?

Numerous scientific studies show that treatment helps many people get and stay sober, reduce alcohol or drug use, and improve their lives. A recent study by Dr. John Kelly and colleagues shows that over 22 million people (who overcame an SUD) report that they no longer have a substance problem. While many of these individuals changed on their own without help from professionals or peers in mutual support programs (usually those individuals with less severe forms of an SUD), 54% benefited from participation in a mutual support program, treatment, or both. Mutual support programs were used by 45%, professional treatment was used by 28%, and medications (for opioid or alcohol addiction) were used by 9%. These results show there are many paths to recovery, and people with the more severe forms of an SUD often respond to professional treatment.

Large surveys of individuals in recovery from an SUD in the United States, Canada, Australia, and the United Kingdom also document many positive effects of treatment and recovery. For example, a survey of recovery in the United States reported by Dr. Alexandre Laudet found that addiction was present for an average of 18 years and caused many problems for the individual and family. Dr. Laudet reported high rates of use of professional treatment (71%), 12-step recovery programs (95%), other mutual support programs (22%), and MAT (18%). Involvement in these services contributed to dramatic improvements in all areas of life, such as:

- Family relationships and reduction of violence
- Use of mental health services for those in need of psychiatric care
- Employment, job training, education, or starting a business
- Financial behaviors such as paying bills, debts, and taxes, and saving for the future
- Community involvement such as volunteer work or voting
- Engaging in healthy behaviors such as taking care of health, more exercise, or better diet.

Other areas include much less use of emergency department services; more enrollment in healthcare benefits; and reduction of illegal acts, incarceration, and involvement in the criminal justice system.

To benefit from treatment, your loved one should:

- Keep all appointments and stay in treatment and/or recovery services long enough to benefit. Dropping out early is usually a bad sign and often precedes relapse.
- Follow through with the agreements made with the counselor or treatment group.
- Use positive coping strategies to deal with the challenges of recovery from an SUD such as resisting pressure from others to use substances, engaging in enjoyable activities to reduce boredom, and increasing involvement in normal family functions.
- Get active in AA, NA, or other mutual support recovery program. Those who become active in 12-step programs, for

example, do better than those who do not attend or who do not use the tools of recovery in their lives.

- Consider other mutual support programs, chatrooms, or recovery clubs as sources of recovery support.

PERSONAL REFLECTION: IT'S NEVER TOO LATE TO GET HELP

There was a time in my life when I thought my dad would never address his severe alcohol problem. I believed he would die as a result of an accident or medical complication. Then, at age 66, he decided to get help during the period my mother was dying of cancer. After my mother's death, my father went to a residential rehabilitation program but left early as he did not feel it was helping him. Later, I connected him with a friend and colleague of mine, an addiction psychiatrist, who evaluated my father and provided ongoing treatment. My dad drove nearly 90 miles each way to see this psychiatrist, who helped him establish and maintain abstinence and reduce anxiety and depression symptoms that were persistent and probably lifelong. My dad occasionally went to local AA meetings when another family member in recovery took him. He lived abstinent from alcohol from age 66 until he died at age 80. Reviewing his extensive history of an alcohol use disorder and how he turned his life around shows that people with severe problems can recover. Both authors of this book know of many people who have had multiple episodes of treatment only to go back to using and then eventually sustaining their recovery over long periods of time. It is hard to predict who will do this or when they will do this, as there are many people motivated to change who use again. So, we say to you: Never give up on your family member. Never lose hope. You can help. Let others help and support you. Positive change may happen some day with your loved one.

6

Recovery from a Substance Use Disorder

WHO WE ARE

- *Bridget got help with her drinking problem from a counselor and by attending Women for Sobriety meetings.* She has been abstinent for over a year. Her family is pleased that she attends family functions without drinking. She visits her parents each week and helps them with tasks around the house. Bridget walks regularly with a friend to stay in shape and keep her weight down.
- *Mitchell was in and out of several rehabs for heroin addiction.* He also went to a methadone clinic but quit after a year. Mitchell overdosed on drugs twice and had to be saved by paramedics. His periods of recovery ranged from a few months to over a year. Mitchell now believes the best path to long-term recovery is counseling, NA meetings, and consistently taking the medication naltrexone (Vivitrol) as a monthly injection. This plan has enabled him to stay drug free and to work on his fractured marriage. Mitchell sometimes brings his wife and son to counseling sessions. He worked with an NA sponsor to make amends to his wife and son for the heartache he caused. Mitchell now feels confident that he can remain drug free. He is active in his son's school and in community activities. Mitchell

    rediscovered the joy of sports with his son. He found that normal family events bring satisfaction and meaning to his life.

- *When Paula quit drugs, she joined a church group.* Even though this group is not designed for drug problems, Paula believes her connection to others, and getting more active in her religion, has helped her stay sober and find meaning in her life.
- *Emilio had trouble staying abstinent while attending outpatient counseling, so he agreed to attend a rehab program to jumpstart his recovery.* After finishing this program (his second rehab stay), Emilio agreed to continue in outpatient treatment and to begin a trial of naltrexone (Vivitrol) to help him control his cravings for alcohol. Emilio also attends AA and has abstained from alcohol for nearly a year. He manages what he calls "my alcoholic thinking" and does not give in to strong urges to drink.

As these examples show, there are many paths to recovery. People with more severe problems may require professional help. Those addicted to opioids or alcohol may also benefit from medications to help sustain recovery. Given his history of relapses, Mitchell would have had trouble sustaining recovery were it not for taking medication for his heroin addiction. Emilio also benefitted from medication for his alcohol problem. Mitchell is much more likely than Emilio to take medication for a longer period of time due to the severity of Mitchell's opioid addiction. Some people, like Paula, were able to quit with no professional help. Usually, though not always, these are people whose problems are in the mild to moderate range. Many benefit from programs like AA or NA, Women for Sobriety, SMART Recovery, LifeRing Secular Recovery, or others.

    Recovery refers to everything that your family member with the SUD does to manage the problem and make positive changes. *Abstinence* is a first step for those who choose this goal, but the real work of recovery is staying abstinent over time *and* making personal changes to support this. Recovery is not short term; it is a process that takes place over years for many people with SUDs.

PATHS TO RECOVERY

Not all people with an SUD work a program of recovery. Some change without the help of professionals or peers in mutual support programs. They use the support of family, friends, and others, or participate in spiritual or religious activities. Individuals with more severe types of SUDs often need professional help and/or participation in mutual support programs to be successful in recovery. The path your family member follows will be based on the severity of the SUD, degree of damage caused by it, her motivation for change, whether another type of SUD or psychiatric disorder is present, support from others, and the availability of recovery resources (professionals and mutual support programs). Potential areas of recovery include:

- *Physical and lifestyle*: improving medical and dental health, exercising, good nutrition, sufficient rest and sleep, and managing substance cravings. Reducing triggers at home such as getting rid of drug paraphernalia can aid recovery
- *Psychological*: accepting the SUD, developing positive attitudes, thinking differently, managing stress and moods, and using active coping strategies
- *Family*: assessing the impact of the SUD on the family and members, involving the family in treatment and recovery, and making amends to others hurt by the SUD. For parents with an addiction, the impact of SUDs on their children should be considered as well as steps to help children deal with the effects of the SUDs
- *Social*: establishing a recovery network with supportive people, refusing substance offers, and engaging in healthy leisure activities. Healthy relationships and mutual support programs are the cornerstone of recovery for many people
- *Spiritual*: overcoming guilt and shame, finding meaning in life, using a higher power, forgiving oneself and others, and helping others or giving back

- *Financial:* dealing with money problems caused or worsened by the SUD; learning to manage a budget wisely; and paying bills, debts, and taxes
- *Other:* addressing and resolving school, work, housing, and legal issues

BENEFITS OF RECOVERY

Recovery is not easy because it forces the person to face problems and adjust to a new way of living. Recovery offers many benefits, however, including the chance for personal growth. Some benefits occur as soon as one stops using alcohol or drugs, while others take time and effort. Some benefits are small, and others are significant. Benefits of recovery are both short and long term. Surveys of individuals in recovery in the United States, Canada, Australia, and the United Kingdom show that large numbers of people are doing well in recovery. In Chapter 5, we listed improvements documented by those who completed the US survey.

People who are impatient and impulsive and want immediate results have difficulty seeing the long-term benefits of recovery and want the benefits now. Don't become discouraged if you see this reaction in your family member—it is common early in recovery. As people with SUDs move through recovery, they learn that progress may be slow and gradual, and that they have to work hard if they are to enjoy the benefits of recovery. Nothing is achieved without working for it.

Some people do not engage in counseling or mutual support programs, and they rely mainly on medication for their recovery from opioid addiction. For example, Alan was addicted to prescription opioids originally prescribed for pain. Although he attended several rehabilitation programs, he was not interested in recovery or attending mutual support programs. All he wanted was medication to help him "stay off opioids." He is not using anymore, and his family relationships have improved as a result.

7

Relapse After a Period of Recovery

WHO WE ARE

- *Brian is a 40-year-old, employed, married father of 2 children, with a 10-year history of alcohol use disorder with multiple treatment episodes.* After he finished a short-term rehab program, Brian attended outpatient counseling. He included his family in treatment sessions and was active in AA. Brian was not drinking for nearly 2 years when he relapsed after he stopped attending AA meetings due to his busy work schedule. His wife insisted he go back to treatment; otherwise she would take the children and move out. He reconnected with his AA sponsor and started outpatient counseling. Brian now has several months of not drinking under his belt. He feels that his wife was instrumental in his getting back into treatment and AA. She goes to some counseling sessions with him, and to Al-Anon meetings.
- *Sarah is a 35-year-old divorced woman with a long history of depression and an opioid use disorder.* Her depression was treated with antidepressant medications and outpatient counseling. This counseling and NA helped her manage her opioid addiction. After being in recovery from using opioids for several years, Sarah got a tooth extracted. He dentist gave her opioids for pain,

and she thought that taking them for a short period of time would not be a big deal. The pain was severe, and Sarah used a 7-day supply in 4 days. She then had strong cravings for opioids. Fortunately her counselor and NA sponsor helped her just when she was about to get more pain pills.

As these examples show, relapse or the possibility of a relapse is always present. Resumed use after a period of recovery and following treatment should not be viewed negatively or in a judgmental way. Rather, relapse is an expectation—not an exception—for people who struggle with SUDs and other medical and chronic conditions. Relapse can happen even after a long period of recovery, as it did with Brian. Although the odds of a relapse decrease the longer a person is not using, there is always a possibility that relapse can happen, even among individuals who are highly motivated to recover. Brian was doing well in his recovery, but he let up on his AA meetings due to being busy with work. This shows that regardless of how long a person is sober, he must be vigilant about recovery. Brian's case also shows that the family can influence the person who relapses to reengage in treatment, which can limit the damage that a relapse can cause.

Sarah's case shows that use of an opioid medication for pain can trigger a desire for more drugs and influence the person to continue using prescription opioids, or in some cases to seek illicit drugs like heroin. By sharing her drug craving with her counselor and NA sponsor, and not keeping it a secret, Sarah was able to get help and support that enabled her to continue recovery without going back to drug use.

LAPSE AND RELAPSE

Using alcohol or drugs after a period of recovery is called a lapse or a relapse. A *lapse* refers to the first episode of use; it may or may not lead to a relapse. Some people prevent a lapse from leading to a relapse. It is hard to predict what may happen when a person lapses. A *relapse* refers to a continued use of alcohol or drugs after the initial lapse. Relapses vary.

Some people get heavily into alcohol or other drugs and experience very negative effects, including death in some cases. Others cut down on the frequency or quantity of use. Some control and limit their use of alcohol or other drugs, but it later gets out of control. When individuals with SUDs start using again and their use does not get out of hand at first, they may believe they can use "socially" or control their use. Some believe they no longer need help from professionals or peers in mutual support programs.

People with SUDs may lapse or relapse only once, several times, or many times. Although it is possible for anyone to get and stay sober, some people are at greater risk for relapse. It is best to view these people as struggling more than others who do better. Think about it: Logically it makes no sense why someone would go back to using substances when this has caused serious problems, yet this happens all the time. Those who relapse are not "bad" but "vulnerable" people who have trouble control-ling their use.

Not only will lapses and relapses vary in frequency or severity, so will their consequences. In some cases, individuals who lapse or relapse be-come more motivated and work harder at recovery. Some stop the lapse or relapse early and avoid major damage. Others experience serious negative consequences as a result. Tragically, some die from a relapse.

The challenge for people in recovery is to be vigilant about relapse and have a plan to catch warning signs and manage high-risk situations or factors to reduce the chances of using again. If they use, the challenge is to stop quickly and limit the damage.

Families may worry about relapse even when their loved one with the SUD is doing well. One of our surveys identified relapse as the second most common concern after drug overdose among family members. The more you know about lapse and relapse, the more supportive and realistic you can be with your family member. Relapsing does not have to be the end of the world; many people learn from relapses and get back on track. You should ask to be part of any discussion of a relapse prevention plan if your relative is in treatment; families often notice warning signs ahead of the person with the SUD.

WARNING SIGNS OF RELAPSE

The risk of relapse is greatest during the first year of recovery, especially the first 3 months. Your loved one is adjusting to being and living substance free. Her brain is also adjusting to being substance free. It may take a long time for her brain to normalize and for her to have fewer and less severe cravings or desires to drink or use drugs. When your family member has strong desires to get high, she is at increased risk for relapse. Don't be too alarmed, as these desires or cravings are common in early recovery. The key is whether your loved one uses coping strategies and social support to fight them off. For example, talking about cravings with a counselor, with peers in recovery, or at mutual support meetings can help the person maintain recovery rather than give in to a craving to use. Or, the person with the SUD can use self-talk strategies to resist the craving (e.g., "even though I want to use, I don't have to; if I wait this out, my drug craving will pass; ain't no way I'm giving in to this craving").

As mentioned in the "Lapse and Relapse" section, relapse refers to using alcohol or drugs after a period of abstinence. The process may start before actual substance use and may show in your loved one's return to old habits and behaviors that increase relapse risk. Sometimes, the relapse pro-cess is obvious, such as when Rosa has a substantial increase in thoughts about drinking or wants to socialize with friends who get together for a few drinks after work. Other times, it is hidden, and the person or family members do not see it happening at first, such as when Zach cuts down on his daily meditation, review of his day, reading recovery literature, or socializing with peers after NA meetings. This is why people with SUDs are encouraged to get involved in long-term recovery.

Experts have identified warning signs or clues that may precede relapse. The late Dr. G. Alan Marlatt wrote about seemingly "irrelevant decisions" that lead to relapse. Usually, using alcohol or drugs is the last link in a chain of decisions. For example, your loved one may cut down on or stop attending counseling sessions or mutual support meetings, weeks or months before a relapse. Or he may reconnect with a friend with whom he previously used and not believe consciously that he wants to use again.

If you ever returned to smoking after quitting or gained weight after breaking a diet, think about the time in which you took the first puff or ate that first piece of cake. This step probably didn't come out of the blue. Most likely, you thought about smoking or breaking your diet, or put yourself at higher risk by decisions you made *before* you relapsed, such as joining coworkers who go on smoke break without the intent of smoking, or buying sweets so you have them in case others come to your house, even though it is hard to resist if you have easy access to eating these sweets.

Many people prevent relapses by catching early warning signs such as changes in attitudes, behaviors, thinking, or moods that indicate a movement toward relapse. As a family member, you can support the person in recovery by pointing out changes that could indicate a potential relapse is on the horizon.

Those who relapse can learn from the experience by reviewing:

- what led up to it
- the early warning signs
- how much time elapsed between these signs and using alcohol or drugs
- where and when the relapse occurred
- who else was present.

Understanding the answers to these questions makes the person better prepared to identify and manage future warning signs *before* using alcohol or drugs. If you share any warning signs that you observe, this may help your family member learn from the relapse.

WHY DO PEOPLE RELAPSE AND USE AGAIN?

Although a solid recovery plan and positive attitude reduce the likelihood of relapse, it can happen with people who think they are immune from relapse or fail to be vigilant in recovery. Relapse usually results from a combination of factors rather than from just one. In some cases, what seems to cause a relapse may be the "straw that broke the camel's back."

Research has identified high-risk factors associated with relapse. People with SUDs are prone to problems like everyone else. In some instances, their response to problems is to use substances. Using in response to an upsetting emotional state or a stressful situation is a quick fix and is easier than devising and using a more time-consuming plan.

Some individuals relapse after receiving medications for a medical or dental problem because this reawakens their desire for drugs. This can take people by surprise if they do not anticipate that it can happen. Individuals in recovery can tell any physician or dentist prescribing addictive drugs that they are in recovery from an SUD.

High-risk relapse factors vary, and most fall into the categories below. *However, it is not the high-risk factor that leads to relapse but the failure to use coping skills to prevent it.*

1. *Failure to manage negative emotions:* shame, anger, anxiety, boredom, depression, loneliness, guilt, or feeling empty or like nothing matters
2. *Positive emotions:* feeling good and believing the SUD is under control, or that a reward is in order
3. *Social influences:* social pressures to use, failure to refuse pressures to use in situations where drugs or alcohol are offered by others, or living with others who have substance problems
4. *Negative thinking:* not fighting off thoughts that contribute to relapse like "relapse can't happen to me; I can control my use; one or a few won't hurt"
5. *Painful memories:* related to mental, physical, or sexual abuse or the loss of a relationship that causes anger, grief, or depression
6. *Family or relationship problems:* conflicts with others, lack of support, involvement with other people with an SUD
7. *Family "sabotage":* lack of support or persistent hostility from family members, or pressure to use from a family member who uses alcohol or drugs

8. *Inability to manage cravings or desires:* not using strategies to manage desires, cravings, or compulsions. Cravings can occur after receiving prescription drugs for a medical problem such as pain. They can also occur after seeing (drug paraphernalia or alcohol), hearing (music associated with getting high), or smelling (marijuana or tobacco smoke) stimuli associated with past substance use.

9. *Psychiatric problems that are not diagnosed or adequately treated:* these may include a mood, anxiety, eating, psychotic, personality, or other type of disorder.

10. *Not catching changes in motivation early:* desires to change can vary from one day to the next. Motivation struggles may show in cutting down or stopping counseling, mutual support meetings, or working a daily plan of recovery.

11. *Problems with self-confidence:* lack of confidence in one's ability to stay sober or being too confident and not remaining vigilant. This can lead to becoming lax in following a recovery plan or using the help and support of others.

12. *Lack of productive roles:* stress caused by not working, or not being involved in roles or activities that bring satisfaction or a feeling of being productive.

13. *Lack of balanced lifestyle:* a lack of routine or structure, too many demands or obligations, or lack of satisfaction with current life.

Relapse factors can be addressed with a plan of personal and lifestyle change. Involvement in counseling and/or mutual support programs helps reduce your loved one's relapse risk.

HELPING AND SUPPORTING YOUR FAMILY MEMBER

While it is not your responsibility to make sure your family member with an SUD does not relapse, you can provide support and help. You don't have to sit back passively and watch him slide back to drinking or using drugs. Here are some strategies to consider:

1. *Let go of your fears of relapse:* you can worry until you are blue in the face and it still won't make a difference to your family member. Use the 12 steps of Al-Anon or Nar-Anon or repeat slogans such as "Let go and let God" to let go of your fears.

2. *Discuss relapse with your family member:* accept that relapse can occur even if your family discusses it. Your family may first have a discussion about the possibility of relapse, or discuss it with a counselor or other families in recovery before talking with the member who has the SUD.

3. *Share your observations of warning signs:* tell your loved one that you want to support her recovery and discuss any relapse warning signs you notice. Tell her your intent is to help reduce her relapse risk, not nag or check up on her. Ask your family member what she wants you to do if you notice relapse warning signs. Be as specific as you can when discussing how to help her by sharing your observations of warning signs.

4. *Develop an emergency plan to deal with a relapse*: discuss what steps to take if your loved one relapses. If you prepare ahead of time, you may feel a greater sense of control if it actually occurs. The earlier a relapse is caught, the greater the likelihood that it can be cut off. If it leads to physical addiction, help your family member get help to determine if detoxification or other treatment is needed.

5. *Review the relapse experience:* talk about your reactions to your relative's relapse when it has ended and he is back on the road to recovery. Don't deny your feelings. If you are upset and angry, then face it. Let him know how you were feeling.

6. *Seek support from Al-Anon, Nar-Anon, or another family support program:* discuss your feelings with a support group, and find out how others deal with their family members' relapses. Members of such groups can listen to your experiences and

feelings as well as share helpful ideas on how to survive a loved one's relapse. You may learn ways to reduce your upset feelings and accept your limitations.

7. *Don't lose track of your own recovery:* keep in mind that there are limits to what you can do to help your loved one if he relapses. Do not let this experience make you lose focus on yourself or on your own recovery. Keep working your program so that you maintain control over your emotions and behaviors.

8. *Consider counseling or therapy:* therapy can help you and other family members understand and support the member who relapsed. You will learn what you can do and what not do to help your loved one. This information can help you or other family members deal with personal reactions to your loved one's relapse. SUDs can bring out the worst in us, so learning to manage our own reactions is just as important as helping our family member with the SUD. If you have an adolescent with an SUD, family treatment is usually the recommended approach.

8

Psychiatric Illness Co-occurring with a Substance Use Problem

WHO WE ARE

- *Will has suffered from multiple episodes of recurrent major depression.* He does well when he is active in mental health treatment and taking his medications. Prior to his last episode of depression, Will went on a cocaine binge and became depressed and suicidal, leading to a psychiatric hospitalization. During this stay, he admitted to his drug problem and agreed to focus both on this and his depression to establish stable recovery. Will has now been drug free for over a year and is in recovery from his depression and cocaine addiction. His parents and partner are relieved and pleased with his commitment to recovery. They attend some counseling sessions with him. His partner attends Nar-Anon when Will goes to NA meetings.

- *Jenna sought treatment for her anxiety and agoraphobic disorders and alcohol use disorder, but had problems initially getting the help she needed.* When she called to arrange for mental health services, Jenna was told to take care of her alcohol problem first. When she called addiction programs, she was told to take care of her mental health problems first. Finally, she found a program that provided treatment for both disorders. This enabled Jenna to establish a relationship with a team that provided integrated care for her disorders. She also returned to AA as this had helped her stay sober in the past. Jenna is now stable and doing much better. Her adult son Brad attended some treatment sessions with his mom, as well as joining a family support group. He feels he has learned some practical tools for dealing with his own worries about his mother.

HAVING BOTH AN SUD AND A PSYCHIATRIC DISORDER

The combination of an SUD and a psychiatric disorder is called dual or co-occurring disorders (CODs). Many community and clinical studies show high rates of CODs. Rates of SUDs are especially high among individuals with antisocial or borderline personality disorders, bipolar illness, and schizophrenia. Having one disorder raises the risk of having the other. Compared to individuals with only one type of disorder, individuals with CODs are more likely to miss treatment sessions, stop treatment early, and not take medications as prescribed. They have more medical and social problems, and they are at higher risk to return to the hospital.

Psychiatric illness can affect (1) how quickly a substance problem develops and (2) response to treatment. It can also affect relapse to substance use. Our studies show that since people with CODs are at risk to drop out of treatment early, this puts them at higher risk for relapse.

The effects of alcohol or other drugs can cause or worsen psychiatric symptoms. For instance, alcohol, sedatives, and opioids can contribute to depression. Many people who are addicted to cocaine, methamphetamine, and other stimulants "crash" into depression following a binge episode, which can create significant disruptions in the circuitry of the brain and the neurochemicals such as dopamine and norepinephrine, thereby affecting mood, motivation, thinking, and cognitive functions. Phencyclidine (PCP), hallucinogens, or chronic stimulant use can cause psychotic symptoms. Psychiatric symptoms caused by the effects of substances may clear up once alcohol and drug use is stopped.

Many people experience depression and anxiety as a result of problems caused or worsened by their SUDs. Some cases of depression are associated with loss of relationships, jobs, dignity, or self-esteem. Sometimes, a relapse to substance use following a sustained period of recovery causes depression. The person feels guilty and shameful, which in turn can cause depression. Depression or anxiety also can be experienced independent of the SUD.

Since alcohol and drugs can mask, trigger, or worsen psychiatric symptoms, it is not always easy to tell which came first, the substance use or the psychiatric disorder. For individuals with long histories of these disorders, the symptoms and problems become so intertwined that it is difficult to determine which came first.

SUDs and psychiatric problems are not always linked, however. Some people are in remission from their psychiatric disorder, then later develop an SUD, and others are in remission from an SUD, and then develop a psychiatric disorder.

PSYCHIATRIC EMERGENCIES

An emergency can occur regardless of your loved one's motivation for change or participation in treatment. Examples of emergencies include the person:

- Being seriously out of touch with reality (e.g., hallucinations or delusions)
- Being unable to take care of basic needs for food, shelter, or protection
- Feeling extremely anxious or fearful, or controlled by obsessions or compulsions
- Being severely depressed, manic, or out of control with behaviors
- Making a suicidal threat, having a plan, or making an actual attempt
- Threatening to hurt or actually hurting another person

Call a psychiatric hospital, crisis center, outpatient clinic, or mental health professional for help if you are concerned about your loved one's mental condition. Some cases may require taking steps to have your loved one legally committed to a psychiatric hospital for an evaluation and treatment. You can even call 911 and ask for help.

SUICIDE

The risk of suicide increases when SUDs and psychiatric illness co-occur. Substances can impair judgment, leading the person to make a suicide attempt. Suicide risk factors include when the person:

- has made a previous attempt
- has an actual plan
- is depressed
- feels hopeless
- has access to firearms
- is suffering a recent loss of someone important, a job, or health

When a loved one talks about suicide, take it seriously. Listen and be supportive. Encourage him to get professional help. Psychiatric hospitalization may be needed if an attempt is threatened or has been made. You may have to initiate an involuntary commitment to get your family member help. Even though it can be uncomfortable to do this, it may be necessary to protect your loved one from attempting to take his life.

You can call your county mental health administration office, a mental health clinic, or a psychiatric hospital for more information about the process of commitment. If your family member is in treatment, you can inform his doctor or therapist of the suicidal talk or behavior. The doctor or therapist can then help you determine the best course of action for your loved one in crisis.

TREATMENT OF CO-OCCURRING PSYCHIATRIC DISORDERS

There are many treatment services for individuals with SUDs who have a co-occurring psychiatric illness. In cases of severe, acute symptoms, psychiatric hospitalization may be needed to help stabilize the person. Other services may include partial hospitalization, intensive outpatient, psychiatric rehabilitation, co-occurring disorders rehabilitation, case management, peer support, and medications. Integrated treatment that addresses both substance use and psychiatric disorders is preferred. This means that your family member would get help for both disorders in the same program by the same treatment team. It is referred to as providing integrated care. However, be prepared that a mental health system or professional may not offer integrated care. Not all mental health practitioners have the knowledge, skills, or comfort level needed to address both types of disorders. Similarly, addiction treatment systems may not be able to adequately treat the psychiatric disorder as practitioners may not have adequate training.

9

How Substance Problems Affect the Family Unit

This chapter will help you understand how families, concerned others, and friends are affected by a loved one's SUD. While not everyone is affected in the same way, many people experience negative effects. The case that follows shows how Trevor's family experienced his wife's SUD. As you read this, think about how your family has been affected by your loved one's SUD.

> *My wife, Brittany, got in serious trouble with cocaine a couple of years ago. A few times, I got her to agree to stop using drugs. The truth is that she told me what I wanted to hear. She never stopped using cocaine even though I thought she did. Brittany was good at fooling me, and I was good at being fooled. I wanted to believe she would stop using drugs so I let myself be deceived. She even took money from our savings and retirement accounts to buy drugs.*
>
> *As things got worse, the kids and I saw less and less of her. Brittany was always on the go and didn't have much interest in being with us. Our children were devastated. Kristin, our 14-year-old, took it very personally that her mom didn't spend much time with her anymore, and Drew, our 11-year-old, was scared that his mom might get hurt in an accident. He was really sad because of what his mom was doing.*

Most of my energy went to taking care of the kids and trying to protect them. We all felt awful and hoped that things would get better. Little did we know at the time, but Brittany was getting worse. When I finally told her to get help or I would take the children and leave, she broke down and agreed.

Even though Brittany was the one using drugs, every one of us suffered. Thank God she's off drugs and in recovery now. The kids and I also attend some sessions with her, and I go to a local family support program.

This scenario shows how Brittany wreaked havoc on her family. Her husband, Trevor, and their children were devastated about their unraveling family situation until Brittany finally got help. Trevor wisely made sure he and the children attended some sessions with her. He also engaged in a family mutual support program.

EFFECTS ON THE FAMILY UNIT

Any family member may be hurt by a loved one with an SUD. The effects may vary among families and among members within the same family, but emotional pain and disruption of family life are common. Attention often centers on the member with the SUD, while overall family pain and distress are ignored.

A family unit is a system in which various parts have an impact on other parts. When one person in the family is impaired, it affects the others. For example, if a parent is suffering from a medical or psychiatric illness, this can upset the balance of the family. Some family members may be upset or worried. Others may take on the responsibilities of the sick person.

The same holds true for a family system in which a member has an SUD. Individuals with SUDs often "underfunction," which means that other members of the family have to pick up the slack and "overfunction." This dynamic may change how family members communicate or relate to one another. Any area of family life can be affected in positive or negative ways. In some families, chaos becomes common. The problem becomes a central focus of family life. They talk about it a lot, and often plan activities or change plans based on the behavior of the person with the SUD. The following comments by family members convey family pain:

- *"Everyone yelled and argued all the time. We were all mad as hell at mom for drinking so much, but took out our frustrations on each other."*
- *"Mom left dad many times, which worried us kids. We didn't know where she went or if she would return. When she finally came back home, it was expected that we act like nothing happened. This was bizarre but the way our family coped."*
- *"My dad's drug use ruined our family. We moved a lot and lived in public housing. Dad couldn't hold jobs so we depended on welfare. I felt ashamed."*
- *"I was mom's sounding board. She complained about my dad's drinking. I felt like a parent to my young sisters as mom was preoccupied with dad's problem."*
- *"Our family never took a vacation and seldom did things together. We went in different directions. Holidays and special occasion were especially bad times because both of my parents drank too much."*

During a 2-week period, I received 7 phone calls or emails from people who were worried or distraught about a family member with an SUD. One contact was from a mother who sent me an email in desperation in the middle of the night, not knowing what to do with her son who was struggling with an SUD and a psychiatric illness. Another was a call from a wife who reported her husband was missing on a cocaine binge. One call was from a father worried about his adult daughter who was in jail and facing severe consequences related to her addiction. I also communicated with a professor from Russia (referred via email to me by a colleague) who asked for advice in dealing with a 38-year-old daughter with a severe alcohol problem and mood disorder. Despite the fact that this professor did so much to try to help her daughter, she felt she was failing her because her daughter kept relapsing and making bad decisions in hooking up with men who had alcohol problems themselves. In all of these instances, family members were hurt and emotionally distraught, yet they focused on helping their loved one as their main priority.

The effects on families vary from mild to severe—in which a family is torn apart by an SUD. Serious problems may result, including death of the person with addiction, the family breaking up due to an addicted parent's inability to care for the children, or the need for relatives or foster care to take care of children when addicted parents are unable to do this.

The effects on a family or its members are determined by:

- the severity of the SUDs
- the presence of other medical, psychiatric, or social problems
- the behavior of the family member with the SUD
- the availability of support within and outside of the family
- exposure to positive relationships or experiences
- personal characteristics such as resiliency and determination.

WAYS FAMILIES COPE

Families cope with SUDs in both effective and ineffective ways. Effective ways may include talking together about the problem and what steps to take, developing a plan should the member with the SUD refuse to get help, seeking support and help for themselves, or not changing family plans to accommodate the member with the SUD. Ineffective ways of coping may include denying the SUD, minimizing its effects, tolerating inappropriate or harmful behavior, taking over the responsibilities of the member with the SUD, or protecting the affected member from the consequences of substance use. It is not unusual for some families to put up with much pain and suffering. Families mean well when they show "kind" behavior. The problem is that such behavior makes it easier for the member with the SUD to continue using alcohol or drugs.

Areas of the family that may be affected by SUDs include:

- *Family mood or atmosphere:* it can feel tense, anxious, sad, depressing, frustrating, or disappointing. Anger and worry are common.
- *Communication:* too much arguing or yelling, not discussing the SUD or talking too much about it, limited expression of positive thoughts or feelings, or too much negativity or focus on problems
- *Interactions among family members:* less cohesion, too much conflict, or failure of parents to work as a team. Family rituals like eating together, sharing activities, worshipping together, and celebrating holidays or special occasions may be harmed.
- *Neglect or abuse:* substance problems are involved in the majority of child abuse and neglect cases. The risk of violence increases among partners or spouses.
- *Relationships:* relatives or friends may avoid you or you may avoid them. Adults and children may feel embarrassed to bring others into the home. Adult children who live outside the family may seldom visit.
- *Financial condition and lifestyle:* the SUD may lead to financial problems due to money spent on drugs or alcohol, unemployment, or underemployment. In some cases, a family may live in poverty, substandard housing, or a homeless shelter.

There is no scientific evidence that family members of people with SUDs experience more psychological problems than the general population. However, family members do suffer negative consequences. Chapters 11 through 13 provide information about treatment and recovery for family members. This information will help you see options available to you, your family, and your children (if you are a parent). Getting involved in recovery for yourself—not just for your family member with the SUD—gives you the chance to deal with any negative effects that you experience.

PART II

Help for the Family Affected by a Substance Use Disorder

10

How Substance Problems Affect Individual Family Members

WHO WE ARE

- *Twelve-year-old Jamal attended a vigil for families who lost a loved one to addiction and lit a candle in his memory of his father.* Over 130 people attended this vigil, mostly adults. When they heard this young boy say, "I light this candle in memory of my dad who died when I was 3," many became tearful. All losses hurt and are painful, but hearing a boy share the loss of his father to a drug problem was especially moving.

- *Rachael grew up in a family with a father who had a severe alcohol problem and who was often absent from family functions.* Rachael became her mother's confidant and looked after her young siblings. She excelled in school and was well liked by everyone. However, Rachael felt something was missing from her life due to her father's absence.

- *Bernie and Liz are raising their two granddaughters because their daughter and her husband have SUDs and unable to function as parents.* The grandparents felt this step was necessary so that their grandchildren would not be removed by Children and Youth Services due to the parents' inability to care for these young girls.

- *Steve is devastated because his young adult son was sentenced to prison after driving drunk and wrecking his car, which killed a person.* His son was usually well behaved, a good student, an athlete with potential, and not much of a party person. Yet one night, Steve's son drank too much, leading to this tragic accident.
- *Julia covers up for her husband's drug problem as best she can.* She is raising their children essentially alone. This is difficult because of her husband's erratic behavior and obsession with medications. Julia is worn out emotionally and physically, but feels she should keep things stable at home.
- *Suki was so despondent and angry when her husband was active in his addiction that she made a list of "ways to kill my husband."* Although her intent at the time was not to kill him, it was her way of expressing her resentment and frustration. When Suki shared this at a mutual support meeting, other members understood what she meant and how she felt. Fortunately, both Suki and her husband are in recovery and doing much better.

These are common situations in families affected by a loved one with an SUD. There are many other examples we could share to show that heartache and heartbreak are found everywhere. Parents, grandparents, spouses, children of all ages, siblings, other relatives, and close friends can be affected in negative ways by a relative's substance problem. Losses are common, both during the active phase of an SUD and after separation; divorce; incarceration; or death from a drug overdose, accident, or medical condition caused or worsened by the SUD.

FAMILY MEMBERS AND SUDs

The effects of SUDs on family members are well documented by researchers, surveys of Al-Anon members, counselors, and people who attend family mutual support programs. Usually, a combination of negative and positive effects is experienced. Some people grow stronger through exposure to an

SUD in their family despite negative effects. They show resilience. Many family members help others in the family who are affected by a loved one's SUD by sharing their stories, educating professionals, and providing help and support in mutual support programs.

It is not easy to establish the relationship between a loved one's SUD and the effects on a given family member. Some problems thought to be caused by SUDs may eventually have occurred in the family even if the SUD did not exist. For example, a child may feel ignored by parent with an SUD who is often absent from the home. Yet this pattern of being absent could still exist even if the parent didn't have a substance problem.

There is evidence that children of parents with an SUD are at higher risk for problems than are children whose parents do not have an SUD. Problems include those related to substance use, health or mental health, trouble with the law, and problems at work or in school.

Any family member can be affected, and the actual effects may vary from one person to another. In one case the negative effects may be quite profound, whereas in another case the effects may be minimal. Even within the same family, members can have a different experience in regard to a loved one's SUD. For example:

Mike and Jim both were exposed to their father's alcohol use during their childhood. Their father, George, was a binge drinker who was intoxicated most weekends. George sometimes was obnoxious and nasty. He said and did many things over the years that hurt Mike and Jim. Mike is still angry, bitter, and upset and feels cheated out of a "normal" childhood. As a kid, he got into trouble with the law, often used drugs and alcohol himself, and dropped out of school early. Mike, age 32, still feels his life is affected too much by what happened during his childhood.

Jim, age 29, does not harbor ill feelings toward his father. Although Jim states he also felt cheated of many things as a child, he has left this all behind and cannot let what happened in the past drag him down. During his teen and young adult years, Jim did not experience the problems his brother did. Jim felt motivated to get ahead. He did not

*want his own family to live in the same chaotic way in which he did as
a child.*

In this situation, two brothers from the same family report different effects
from growing up in a family with a father with an alcohol problem. One
brother (Jim) was more resilient than the other.

PROTECTIVE FACTORS AND RESILIENCE

Dr. Robert Ackerman has written about effects of SUDs on families and
children as well as offsetting or protective factors. He believes that not all
young or adult children are affected in the same way by a parent's SUD.
Protective or offsetting factors may be internal and relate to a family
member's beliefs, perceptions, abilities, talents, or personality. Some of
us are more prone to stress than others. And some of us are more resilient than others and are able to tolerate or bounce back from difficult
experiences because of our coping skills.

Offsetting factors include supportive relationships and other influences.
Aisha, who grew up with a mother with a drug addiction, stated that
she directed time and energy to music. She also benefited from the attention and compassion of her music teachers whom she looked up to
as role models. Aisha believes that these mentors helped her survive a
difficult time.

Some family members make the best of the situation, using their
strengths to help themselves and other family members. In a book enti-
tled *The Resilient Self,* Drs. Steven and Sybil Wolin describe how survivors
of troubled families, including families affected by SUDs, can rise above
adversity. They say that by using resiliency skills, the family member can
manage painful memories, put the past in its place, stop wishing for all the
scars of the past to go away completely, *and live well in the present.*

The Wolins believe there are two forces at work in troubled families: dangers that can damage the child and challenges that can provide
an opportunity for growth. The Wolins encourage survivors of troubled

families not to get bogged down in the "damage model," where the focus is on the injuries of the past.

IMPACT ON FAMILY MEMBERS, INCLUDING CHILDREN

The Center for Substance Abuse Treatment reported that parental SUDs underlie many family problems such as divorce, spouse abuse, child abuse and neglect, welfare dependence, and criminal behaviors. Studies show that women who use alcohol or drugs during pregnancy are more likely to give birth to babies prematurely. These babies are often born with a lower birth weight and have medical complications requiring more neonatal care. Recent years have seen a significant increase in babies of mothers with opioid addiction born with neonatal abstinence syndrome (NAS). These babies require medical care in a neonatal intensive care unit in a hospital. Babies born to mothers with alcohol addiction may be born with complications as well.

Studies of children of parents with SUDs find that these kids are at higher risk than other kids to develop alcohol, drug, mental health, behavior, or academic problems themselves. Researchers believe that these children experience impairments in the executive functions of the brain, which are areas associated with organizing, planning, reasoning, and problem solving.

We conducted a survey of 140 outpatients in treatment for SUDs and psychiatric disorders. The patients rated the negative effects of both their SUD and their psychiatric illness on their families as "very serious." Specific effects included:

- Emotional burden on family—91%
- Neglecting the family—84%
- Verbal abuse—70%
- Financial hardship—64%
- Physical abuse—45%

- Giving children to relatives or having child welfare agencies take them—37% (of parents)
- Arrested for intimate partner violence—27%

What these statistics do not convey is how family members feel or deal with the negative impact of a loved one's addiction. For example, "emotional burden" for some family members may show in severe clinical depression requiring professional help.

SUDs FROM THE PERSPECTIVE OF THE FAMILY MEMBER

Over the years, the authors have interviewed many family members and individuals with SUDs about their personal experiences. All reported negative effects on the family resulting from the SUDs. Any area of life can be affected, including school, work, social relationships, physical health, and emotional health. Here are comments by family members that convey what it was like for them.

- **Pete:** "My dad's alcoholism messed with me in many ways. I didn't do well in school and almost dropped out. I got in trouble with the law, and I started fights because I was so angry and wanted to punish others for what I'd been through."
- **Shannon:** "I worried about mom all the time. She couldn't cope with dad's drinking. He'd yell, cuss, and hit her. It was embarrassing. I wouldn't bring friends home because I never knew what dad would do."
- **Lorraine:** "I hated the SOB. He didn't do nothing for me or anyone else in the family. He treated my mom like crap."
- **Earlene:** "I still think of what I missed because my mom died of a drug overdose when I was a kid. I can't believe I lost my mother to drugs. It still haunts me."

- **Angela:** "I had to be both mother and father to our kids. No matter how much I gave the kids, they still were deprived because of my husband's drug problem."
- **Ramon:** "I got so tired and worn out I had to leave my marriage. I couldn't fix things by myself although God knows how many times I tried. My wife wouldn't listen to me."
- **Carolyn:** "My non-abusing child was pretty much left alone while energies were focused on putting out fires with the drug-abusing child."
- **Dennis:** "Our son died from complications related to his addiction. He was only 27. I can't believe he isn't here. We are so despondent over losing him."

Years after leaving a family in which an SUD existed, you might still feel pain and hurt. Many family members have shared with us that, even years later, they still feel disappointment, sadness, anger, guilt, shame, worry, or even hatred.

The emotional burden on parents can also be high as they may feel responsible for their child's SUD and wonder what they could have done differently to prevent it. Parents are often heartbroken and can experience any of the awful things that can happen to other family members.

A mother of a young man who died of a heroin overdose once called me and asked if she could donate his body to our medical center to study his brain. She thought this would help our understanding of SUDs. It was one of the ways she was trying to deal with the heartbreak of losing her 26-year-old son to a drug overdose.

Spouses who live with a partner with addiction may feel angry, guilty, depressed, or responsible for the problems in the family caused or worsened by the SUDs. They may focus so much on their partner with addiction that their children do not get the time and attention they need.

> I heard Senator George McGovern share his story of the death of one of his daughters due to her alcoholism. It was a gut-wrenching story that ended with her getting drunk and freezing to death in the snow. She was the mother of young daughters. Senator McGovern shares his family's story in an insightful and moving book entitled *Terry.* His daughter also suffered from depression, so his book gives insight into what Senator McGovern refers to as the "double demons" of "alcoholism" and depression.

Young and adult children, spouses, siblings, and parents show a variety of responses to the SUDs. Although each person's situation is unique, the common denominator among family members is emotional pain and heartache.

Your relationship with your relative with the SUD may contribute to feeling like your life is out of control. Your life may center on this person. Any area of your life can be affected—how you think, feel, and behave; your physical and mental health; your spirituality; and your relationships with others. However, even if your own life is out of control, you may continue trying to control your loved one.

WAYS SUBSTANCE USE CAN AFFECT FAMILY MEMBERS

Next we discuss different ways that SUDs can affect family members. Think about how these apply to you and to other family members, including children (of course, not all of these may apply to you).

Preoccupation with the Member with the SUD

You become overly concerned or preoccupied with the family member. You worry and may center your life around this person whether he is doing poorly or doing well. You become so concerned that you may even lose yourself in the process. Your self-esteem or mood may go up and down, depending on whether your family member is doing well or poorly. Your preoccupation can be present when your family member is using alcohol or other drugs and even when he is doing well in recovery, as you worry about whether a relapse will happen.

Deny or Minimize the Problem

You deny or minimize the SUD or the negative effects of it on the affected person, the family, or yourself. You may deny the SUD because the person doesn't always show signs of using alcohol or drugs, doesn't use every day, or goes to work or functions adequately, or her life doesn't seem to be dominated by alcohol or other drugs. Parents may deny a child's problem with alcohol or other drugs because of the belief that this substance use reflects on them as parents. Or they may think "it's only weed, not a serious drug like cocaine or heroin."

Negative and Positive Reinforcements of Drug Use

Making use easier or reinforcing it is called "enabling" behavior (a term we are not fond of). This may be passive, in which nothing is done and the SUD is accepted and tolerated (*"There's nothing we can do; it's hopeless; he will never stop"*). This may show in observing the person using and not saying anything about it, or not making attempts to get him to seek help. Try to refrain from doing things that make using substances easier for your relative with the SUD. For instance, don't bail him out of trouble, don't pay his bills, and don't give him money. When you do not protect your loved one from negative consequences, he may face the SUD. It is just as important—if not more so—for you to provide positive reinforcement for nonuse, alternatives to use, and healthy behaviors. This may help influence your family member to get help. Clearly, family members can be instrumental in supporting recovery.

Overfunctioning

You may overfunction to make up for what the affected member cannot do. You try to fix the problem, make others in the family feel better, or take over the responsibilities of the person with the SUD. We have seen family members bend over backwards to help out others so often that they focus on taking care of everyone else's needs but their own. Even some young children function like an adult to keep the family going. Family members who focus too much on others, though, may not focus enough on their own health and well-being. Or they may feel guilty or as if they failed if they don't influence the relative with the SUD to get help.

Mental Health

Anxiety, depression, anger, and guilt are common emotions felt by family members. In some cases, these emotions may be symptoms of a psychiatric illness. Many people who seek help for personal problems or psychiatric illness are members of a family or in an intimate or close relationship in which an SUD is a significant problem. The pain associated with such a relationship may contribute to mental health problems such as depression or anxiety.

Abuse, Neglect, and Violence

Alcohol and drug problems are common among parents who abuse or neglect their children. A parent with an SUD is more likely to be absent from the home and neglect the children.

Many studies document increased rates of violence with alcohol or drug use or SUDs. This may occur due to the effects of the substance on the person's judgment and decision making. Or it may occur as a result of being involved in a drug-using culture in which threats and episodes of violence occur for all sorts of reasons—disagreements, failure to pay a drug debt, or robbing others to get money for drugs.

Loss Through Death

A harsh reality is that people die from alcohol or drug overdoses, accidents, injuries, diseases caused or worsened by SUDs, complications associated with withdrawing from alcohol or other drugs, or being the victims of violence. Parents lose adolescent and adult children. Young children and adults lose parents. Brothers and sisters lose siblings. One man came home from school at age 9 and found his dad dead from a drug overdose. Seeing the dead body and losing his father caused him much anguish, which stuck with him for years. An 11-year-old girl in a program for children of parents with SUDs talked about her drawing (the therapist used art to help kids express their feelings). This young, innocent girl said, "Mom hit me, she punched me, she slapped me, but the very worst thing she did was she died."

Physical Health and Substance Use

Your own health can suffer from worrying about your family member with the SUD. You may become depressed; not take care of yourself; not eat properly; or increase your use of cigarettes, alcohol, or other drugs to deal with stress. According to researchers, family members with an SUD in the family use medical resources at higher rates than members of families in which an SUD does not exist. Spouses or partners sometimes report a loss of interest in sex because of the emotional pain experienced. As one wife said, "When you're tired and worn out from worrying so much, you could care less about sex."

Many studies find that children of parents with SUDs have much higher rates of alcohol or drug problems compared to children with parents without SUDs. In some families, SUDs cut across multiple generations.

Relationships

SUDs can be a factor in isolating from friends or social activities. Parents' relationships with their children may suffer. One mother reported that she got angry and upset over her addicted son. She directed much of this anger at her other two children who bore the brunt of her frustrations. We have seen marriages suffer high levels of stress and conflict because the parents argued and fought over how to deal with their son or daughter with SUD.

The effects on relationships can be subtle. These effects may show in problems with intimacy, an inability to stick with a relationship and make a commitment, excessive focus on others, putting your own needs and desires on the back burner, an irrational desire to please others, a tendency to get involved in abusive and negative relationships, an inability to be satisfied with others, or a tendency to be too critical. (Of course, relationship problems are not limited to people exposed to SUDs.)

Despite the pain experienced, it is not unusual to appear to others as though things are fine. This may result from minimizing the seriousness of the problem, or hoping that if you act as if something is OK, it will be OK. Some people do not want to burden others with their personal pain.

Role Reversal

If one parent has an addiction, a child can become a surrogate parent or confidant to other parent. This puts the child in a position in which he has to act older than his age.

If it weren't for me and my older brother helping out my mother financially when we were growing up, our family would have gone without food. We made money in many ways as young as age 10, and we often shared it with mom because she was often flat broke.

Academic

A long-term study compared sons of fathers with drug problems to sons of fathers who did not have drug problems. The sons with fathers who had drug use disorders had higher rates of problems in many areas. This included lower IQ scores and lower school performance. One adult woman who grew up in a family with alcohol addiction said, "Me and all my siblings were underachievers in school. Two of us even dropped out of high school."

I did so poorly in high school that all the colleges and universities I applied to rejected me. I had to start my college career by attending a local community college.

Juvenile Delinquency

Studies show that problems with the law are more common among children with a parent with an addiction. This may result from poor parental supervision, substance use of the child, or the child getting involved with the wrong crowd. Or it can result from failure to learn and internalize certain values or behaviors or a genetic predisposition. Sons whose fathers are addicted and have a history of criminal involvement have higher rates of antisocial behavior and addiction themselves, very similar to their fathers. These sons often start showing these behaviors during their teenage years.

Although we were not "bad" kids, I and most of my siblings were involved in delinquent behaviors; three of us were incarcerated in juvenile or adult criminal justice facilities.

Financial Problems

Financial burdens result from lost income or money spent on alcohol, drugs, or legal problems created by SUDs. One family we worked with was kicked out of several houses and an apartment because they fell behind on paying rent. Both parents were addicted to alcohol and lots of money was squandered on alcohol. Things got so bad after both parents lost their jobs that the family went on public assistance. Their children often went without adequate food or clothing.

I can remember many times when there was little food in the house and watching my mother figure out how to get one meal at a time. I learned to appreciate tea and toast for breakfast and ketchup sandwiches for lunch. Food insecurity was often a way of life for us.

Ron struggled with cocaine addiction and gambling, and he lost all his money and his business. He did not get help until he also lost his house and his wife divorced him. His addictions created considerable resentment, havoc, and instability within his family. Ron engaged in NA and treatment and ended up going back to college at age 45. Once a millionaire, he now works for a modest salary, but feels his life is more satisfying and meaningful. He has reconnected with his adult children, too.

Other Negative Effects

Some family members who have a loved one with an SUD report feeling angry at God. They give up their religious faith or practices. Some lose hope. When the latter happens, it can be a sign of clinical depression that may need treatment from a professional. If you are worried about your family member or are upset and angry, this can affect you at work or school. Tracy, for example, would sometimes be late for work following her husband's drinking binges. They would argue late into the night, and Tracy would have trouble sleeping. She not only came to work late and tired but would be so upset and angry that she had trouble concentrating on her job.

Positive Effects

Not all of the effects of SUDs are negative. Many people use their experiences to help others. Some family members become closer as a result of bonding together to deal with SUDs. Others become driven to work hard and do well in school, athletics, work, or other areas of life.

> I have a friend who lost a son to a drug overdose. My friend opened up several treatment clinics for people with addictions. She used her grief to help others with addiction and their families. I have friends active in family support programs who help others by sharing their experiences, strength, and hope. I attended a meeting one night where the group was providing support to a member unable to attend because he was sitting with his son in the hospital after the son overdosed and was in a coma. The love, support, and encouragement shared was moving.

Some people are more resilient than others. As a result, they are less negatively affected by difficult or stressful situations such as a family member's SUD. Everyone's personality is different, making some people less vulnerable than others to stress and enabling them to cope more effectively with SUDs in the family.

In Chapters 11 through 13 of this guide, we discuss treatment and recovery for family members who are motivated for change. You will learn steps you can take to help yourself and others in your family.

PERSONAL REFLECTION

Every member of my family experienced negative effects of my father's serious and long-term alcohol problem, and he also had mental health problems. Anger, anxiety, and fear were my companions for many years. Academic underachievement and juvenile delinquency were just a few of the "side effects" that I personally experienced.

I feel fortunate that I healed over time, forgave my father, and used my motivation and my resilience to work hard and succeed in life. I think the lessons I learned shaped my character. Despite my early troubles, I feel I became a better, more empathic, and passionate person due to these experiences. And, this played a significant role in my choosing a career involving service to others affected by mental health, addiction, and other serious problems.

11

Treatment and Recovery for the Family

TREATMENT FOR THE FAMILY

As you know from previous chapters, SUDs have many negative effects on families, so treatment provides a way to deal with these effects. Treatment professionals can help you and your family influence your loved one with the SUD to get help. These professionals can assist you and others to cope with the problems created by the SUD, which can result in improved mood, feeling more in control of your life, and being less focused on your family member with the SUD.

Treatment can also introduce you to recovery and mutual support programs like Al-Anon or Nar-Anon. These programs provide support that continues after treatment is finished, helping you continue to grow and change.

Residential Family Treatment Programs

Some residential and hospital-based programs for people with addiction offer residential programs for their family members. These programs last for several days to a week or more and involve participation in lectures, discussions, therapy sessions, and mutual support meetings. While you may attend treatment activities with your family member who has the SUD, you may also attend some activities without him.

Some centers provide a family program regardless of whether or not your affected family member is in treatment. Such programs focus on helping you understand your own issues and gain a greater sense of control over your life.

If your family member is in a rehab program, ask her about family services that are provided. If she gives you the runaround, call the treatment program directly, express your concerns, and inquire about services for families.

Family Education and Support Programs

Residential and hospital-based inpatient programs usually offer these options during weekends or evenings. These are less intense than programs where families stay onsite but can be very educational and supportive.

Outpatient Counseling

Programs, clinics, and private counselors may offer individual, group, or family counseling. Counseling focuses on your concerns for yourself, for your loved one with the SUD, and for other family members, including any children. Many studies show that adolescents and adults improve when they participate in family therapy. This doesn't mean that other treatments can't help, but family therapy may enhance the outcomes of treatment. These therapies can have an impact on stopping or reducing substance use and helping individuals with am SUD and their spouses to become more stable in their relationships, and children often benefit when parents improve.

You can still benefit from help even if your family member with an SUD refuses to attend sessions with you or to get help for the SUD. Remember to take care of yourself.

Assistance Getting Your Loved One into Treatment

An intervention can be used to encourage a family member with an SUD to get treatment, even if she doesn't want help. Some programs and private counselors or recovery coaches offer this service. There are several different approaches to these interventions, most of which show good rates of treatment entry for the person with the SUD. (These programs include Community Reinforcement and Family Training [CRAFT], A Relational Intervention Sequence for Engagement [ARISE], brief strategic family therapy, multisystemic family therapy, and behavioral couples therapy.) Family members often feel or function better when an intervention is attempted even if their relative struggling with an SUD refuses to get help.

RECOVERY OF THE FAMILY

A *system* refers to a combination of parts that work together to form the whole. A family is a complex system with many parts, each of which affects the others. For example, when one family member is sick with a medical, psychiatric, or substance problem, other members of the family are affected. They may feel upset, worried, angry, or responsible. Or they may try to pick up the slack and take over the sick member's responsibilities.

The different parts of a family system are:

- roles assumed by the individual family members
- rules or guidelines governing behavior (usually unspoken and unwritten)
- family relationships and patterns of interacting within the family (e.g., spouse to spouse, spouse to child, child to child)
- relationships with extended family members (e.g., grandparents, aunts, uncles)
- communication patterns
- family rituals

For the overall family, recovery involves changing how the family functions. It not only has to adjust to the sobriety of the recovering member (if this person is in recovery) but also has to make changes to function more effectively as a unit.

Areas the family may need to address include accepting the SUD, stopping behaviors that reinforce substance use, improving communication, shifting family roles, reestablishing boundaries between generations, and building family togetherness. In some families, problems such as violence or abuse must be addressed. Professional treatment may be needed to address these issues and make changes in how the family functions. The change process can continue after treatment in mutual support programs.

Not all families are alike in what need to change. What a family addresses depends on (1) the impact that SUDs has had on the system and (2) what the family wants to change. Some families resist systemic change and think of recovery as relating only to the person with the SUD. This is a natural reaction to SUDs but one that must be challenged. Otherwise, the family may remain focused on the person with addiction and not change how it operates.

In some cases a family member may be in recovery but other members are not interested or not available. Obviously, the entire family system cannot work together to change if some family members have no interest or investment in recovery or are unavailable. In the rest of this chapter, different areas of family recovery are discussed. For family members, recovery involves (1) learning information, (2) overcoming the emotional distress caused by a close relationship with a relative with an SUD, and (3) making personal changes.

WHAT CAN FAMILIES DO?

There are a number of effective strategies that you can follow to help rebuild your family from the negative effects of SUDs. These include:

- Accept the substance problem.
- Don't cover up the problem.

- Improve family communication.
- Reestablish effective family roles.
- Promote family togetherness.
- Stop abuse or violence.
- Seek professional help.

Accept the Substance Problem

The starting point for change in the family system is to acknowledge that an SUD exists and that the family is affected. If family members deny or minimize the SUD or its effects on the family system, changes are not likely to occur. Acceptance requires honesty and a willingness to face the truth about the SUD. The family can discuss the SUD and the details of its impact on the family unit and individual members.

Don't Cover Up the Problem

Don't make excuses for your relative with the SUD, don't shield him from the negative consequences of his substance use, and don't passively accept it and do nothing about it. These behaviors may be motivated by good intentions as the family does what it thinks is best. However, the outcome is the member with the SUD is less likely to do something about the problem if there are no consequences.

The member may have to face the consequences of substance use. For example:

Jerome's cocaine addiction got so bad that he lost his business, his truck, his equipment, and every cent he had. To support his addiction, he started to write bad checks and stole blank checks from his father that he forged and cashed. He wrote thousands of dollars' worth of bad checks. At first, Jerome did a lot of lying and wheeling and dealing to cover his tracks, but things eventually caught up with him. He was arrested and put in jail. Despite Jerome's long history of addiction and prior criminal record, his parents were going to post bond so he could get out of jail. However, they changed their minds.

Had they posted bail for their son, the message Jerome may have gotten might have been, "Don't worry about getting in trouble. Mom and dad will bail you out." Plus, he may have continued to use cocaine since he would have been shielded from negative consequences (going to prison for crimes committed to buy drugs). Interestingly, after being in prison for about a year, Jerome got active in NA. When he left prison, he attended a treatment program and has been drug free for over 10 years.

We believe people with addiction are often put in prison when they could benefit instead from treatment, but the reality is that many people with SUDs will spend time in jails or prisons.

An open discussion among family members can help identify examples of family behaviors that are not helpful in the long run. If you yourself behaved in this way, don't judge yourself harshly: You did what you thought was needed at the time to help your family member with addiction.

Improve Family Communication Skills

Family members can share reactions and feelings to each other's behaviors as they relate to the SUD; depending on the family, the member with the SUD can be present during these discussions or not. This sharing should be done without hostility or contempt. The family member who receives the feedback should not be defensive. If, for example, a mother constantly shields her husband from the negative consequences of his drinking, their children can talk about how this affects them and how they feel about it. The mother should listen to her children's feelings and concerns. If a daughter with an SUD gets most of the time and attention from her parents, the other children in the family should share their reactions and feelings about this.

Open communication can bring the family closer together. It helps members understand each other and establishes the norm that attention should be directed toward all family members. Although it is helpful for the family to openly discuss these issues, by no means should the communication always revolve around the SUD and associated problems. Communication should focus on other experiences, interests, opinions, and ideas of family members. Families should talk about positive experiences and events. They can share accomplishments and the good things they observe or experience themselves. Giving compliments is a helpful strategy to make family members feel good about one another.

Reestablish Effective Family Roles

SUDs cause roles in the family to shift. Family members may take on the responsibilities or roles of the person with the addiction. A child, for example, may end up in a surrogate parent role in which he takes care of brothers and sisters. A child or teen may fall into the trap of becoming a confidant to the parent who does not have an addiction, listening to problems and offering advice and comfort. A parent may assume the roles of both mother and father because the spouse is impaired by the SUD.

Roles that have been assumed by family members may need to change for the family to move toward health. The recovering member may need to reintegrate into the family and assume roles that were avoided or taken over by other members during the active addiction. For example:

When Lonnie got sober, he assumed the roles of responsible husband to his wife and father to his two daughters. He did his share of disciplining and teaching the children rather than letting this fall on his wife's shoulders as had been the case. Lonnie's wife, Rhonda, had to shift her role as chief caregiver and stop trying to function as both mother and father. Their oldest daughter, Laurel, had to shift her role as mom's "best buddy" in which she listened to her mother's complaints about her father's drinking.

Lonnie was able to resume his appropriate roles with little difficulty. However, Rhonda had trouble letting go of her need to control the family. She got jealous of Lonnie and felt threatened by the fact that the children began talking to him about their problems. Initially, she felt angry and unappreciated. Fortunately, Rhonda worked through these issues in treatment, and the family is doing well now with members assuming appropriate roles. Boundaries between parents and the children are now maintained, whereas during Lonnie's active drinking, they had been blurred.

Promote Family Togetherness

One of the benefits of recovery is that the family becomes closer and more cohesive. Family togetherness develops when members communicate openly with each other and share what is going on in their lives. Sharing activities and experiences and attending mutual support programs promotes togetherness.

Developing family routines and rituals also builds family togetherness. Many events, such as birthdays, graduations, and holidays, are ruined by alcohol and drug use. Recovery gives the family an opportunity to reestablish rituals or develop new ones, and enjoy special occasions together.

Stop Abuse or Violence

Emotional, sexual, and physical abuse can be caused or worsened by an SUD. The family should not tolerate any abuse or violence. The effects of exposure to violence on children can be deep and long lasting whether the child is the recipient of violence or an observer. For example, 19-year-old Santiago stated that seeing his mother and sister hurt by his father during drunken rages was more emotionally disturbing to him than the punishments he personally endured when hit by his father.

Similarly, the effects of sexual abuse on children are harmful and can cause emotional damage for a long time. Children need to feel safe in their homes. Abuse has to stop so the child can heal.

Spouses sometimes suffer physical and emotional abuse as well. As a result, they may live in fear and feel victimized by their circumstances. They may feel trapped and not have the psychological or financial resources to stand on their own.

If violence was or is an issue for your family, there should be a plan to follow should abuse or violence occur again. Violence should not be tolerated. When children are in the home, they need to be protected by adults from violence.

Seek Professional Help

Professional help may be needed for the family unit to resolve problems and make changes. This is especially true in cases involving abuse or violence. Any questions or concerns you have can be discussed with a counselor or family therapist. The advice of friends or sponsors in Al-Anon, Nar-Anon, and other support groups can be sought as well.

In the next chapter, recovery of the individual family member is discussed. This will help you focus more on yourself and less on your loved one with an SUD.

12

Recovery for Individual Family Members

It is common to initially get involved in your family member's treatment mainly to support him in getting and staying sober. However, as you start learning about SUDs, recovery, and the impact on family members, you may realize that involvement in your own recovery offers you a chance to address your personal issues, make changes, and grow as a person. Recovery refers to:

- learning about SUDs and their impact on you
- healing from emotional hurts you experienced
- making changes so that you feel better about yourself and more in control of your life.

WHO WE ARE

The following example shows how a 73-year-old mother was able to change. Listen to Sophie's story and see if you can relate to anything she says:

My son, Fred, who is 42 years old, has been an alcoholic for most of his life. After a drinking bout, he went to a hospital for help. The doctors took care of his medical problems and told him he needed treatment

for his alcohol addiction. Fred was able to get into a treatment pro-
gram, and soon after he started his counselor called and asked me and
his stepfather, Phil, to attend a family program. We had many chances
to talk about Fred's drinking problem and how it affected us. We also
talked about how we affected Fred.

I was advised to stop paying Fred's bills and cleaning his apartment.
The counselors and other family members told me I was too protective
of my son. I learned that all the time I spent fixing his problems or
worrying about him upset my husband Phil more than I ever realized.
I hadn't paid much attention to Phil's feelings. Many times he told me
to set limits with Fred, but I didn't listen.

After Fred finished the rehab program, he returned to his apart-
ment. He did well for about 6 months. Then he started drinking
again and begging me for money. I was able to discuss these
problems during Al-Anon meetings, where I gained the strength
and courage to change MY behaviors. I stopped worrying so much
about Fred and started taking more interest in my husband and
my own life.

I refused to pay his bills even when Fred threatened never to call
me again if I didn't give him money to pay his rent. No longer do I feel
responsible for my son or feel that I have to control his life. The more
I tried to control Fred, the less control I had. So I let go of my "mother's
need" to take care of my adult son. I'm there to support him in recovery,
but I refuse to protect him from the consequences of his drinking. My
husband and I get along better now. We talk more openly about how to
handle Fred, and I value Phil's opinion.

This is an example of a mother in recovery who made changes in herself and improved her relationship with her husband. She stopped
reinforcing and protecting her adult son from the consequences of
his drinking. She stopped taking care of his financial responsibilities. Sophie pays more attention to her own needs now and is not
as obsessed with her son's illness. As a result, she feels better about
herself and gets along better with her husband.

RECOVERY FOR THE FAMILY MEMBER

You will be better prepared to change if you view recovery as a process that takes time, effort, and work. You have to go at your own pace. Avoid the trap of expecting too much, too soon. Go slowly and appreciate even the small changes that you make.

Think about what changes you need to make and are willing to make. The goals of recovery are to accept your limitations, deal with the realities of a loved one's SUD, manage your emotions and behaviors, and take care of your needs.

Following is a discussion of areas of change to consider. Use these as guidelines—you do not have to change in all these areas. Discuss your ideas for change with a counselor, sponsor in Al-Anon or Nar-Anon, or a trusted confidant.

Psychological and Behavioral Change

The area of psychological and behavioral change refers to attitudes, how you think, what you feel, and how you act and cope with problems.

- *Accept your limitations.* Although you can influence and help your family member with an SUD, there are limits to what you can do. Your family member is responsible for her own recovery. The harder you try to control, the less control you have. For example, you may influence your family member to seek help by pressuring her into treatment, but what happens in treatment is up to her. Remember the part of the Serenity Prayer that says "accept the things I cannot change."
- *Don't deny the impact of the SUD.* Admit that the SUD affects you and your family. Don't minimize it. Review the ways in which your thinking, emotions, and behaviors are affected. Be mindful that the SUD can impact other family members—you can't control how your loved ones react or are affected, but you

can treat them with understanding, compassion, and empathy. If the SUD causes a rift in the family, there is the possibility of forgiveness and healing.

- *Do not cover up drug use behaviors.* Don't "overprotect" your family member by covering up for his behaviors or by taking on his responsibilities. Let him face the consequences if he refuses to stop. Give positive feedback when he is sober.

- *Convey expectations.* Let your family member know what your expectations are, especially if she lives in your household. You help more by being firm than by giving in to manipulations or selfish demands.

- *Reduce focus on the member with the SUD.* Try not to let your life revolve around your affected member, whether or not he is still using substances. Pay attention to other family members and your own needs. Work on your recovery regardless of what he does.

- *Accept the ups and downs of recovery.* While progress occurs, so do setbacks. When you get hope, find relief, and start learning and changing, it is natural to feel optimistic and good. This may change as you settle into recovery and face problems or setbacks, especially if your loved one has a relapse.

- *Talk about your feelings and emotional pain.* Don't be held an emotional hostage to the family member struggling with an SUD. Acknowledge and share your feelings and pain with others. Letting go of anger, disappointment, sadness, and other feelings paves the way for forgiveness and change. This is an ongoing process as emotional pain takes time to work through. Sharing pain with other members in mutual support groups can be a potent healing force. If you are in counseling, talk about your feelings as a way of release, to increase your self-understanding, and to learn healthy coping strategies.

- *Consider professional treatment if you persistently feel angry, anxious, or depressed.* Therapy can help you work through and cope with your emotional pain. You can seek personal therapy at a mental health clinic or with a private therapist (psychiatrist, psychologist, social worker, or counselor). If your anxiety or depression is severe and part of a psychiatric disorder, interferes with your ability to function, and does not improve enough with therapy, you may benefit from an evaluation for medication by a psychiatrist or other healthcare professional.

- *Acknowledge and use your strengths.* Don't focus only on problems. Even if you feel stressed out, keep in mind that you have strengths that have helped you cope with other difficulties (e.g., social skills, supportive friends, sense of humor, religious beliefs, and ability to persist). Use these strengths to help you cope during difficult times. And be sure to acknowledge your efforts and attempts.

Social and Family Areas of Change

Take a look at your family, social relationships, and activities to figure out if you need to make any changes. Here are some areas of change to consider.

- *Keep up your friendships.* Some people in a family with a loved one with an SUD decrease or stop socializing with others. They get so caught up in the emotional turmoil caused by the SUDs that they keep to themselves. They reduce or stop calling, visiting, or having others visit them. If you have lost touch with friends or family, get back in touch with them by writing, emailing, texting, contacting them on social media, calling, or arranging visits. Stay connected with friends and use them as sources of support.
- *Engage in social activities or hobbies.* A substance problem in your family can affect your interest in fun activities. This in turn may lead to depression. Participate in activities or hobbies that you enjoy. Have activities and hobbies you can do alone or share with others. Do things that bring you joy and that you look forward to.

- *Focus on family members who do not have a substance problem.* The SUD can be so overwhelming that it engulfs you. You may pay less attention to other family members, particularly if they don't show signs of trouble. Take an active interest in what they are doing. Ask how they have been affected by the SUD.

- *Make amends to family or friends who have been hurt by your behavior.* If any of your actions or inactions caused hurt to others, acknowledge this. You can then decide if you need to make amends. For example, in the situation presented earlier in this chapter, Sophie made amends to her husband, Phil, by apologizing for not listening to his opinions of their son's SUD and ignoring Phil as she got too involved with their son. Sophie paid more attention to her husband's needs and spent more time together in activities that he enjoyed. A counselor or a sponsor in Al-Anon or Nar-Anon can help you know when and how to make amends.

- *If you have children, encourage them to talk about their experiences and feelings.* Teach them about SUDs, recovery, and how families and individual members can be affected. Encourage them to talk about what it was like, how they feel, and what they worry about. Use books written for children to aid their understanding and expression of feelings. Take them to some sessions if you are involved in counseling.

Spiritual Issues

The area of spiritual issues involves overcoming guilt and shame, forgiving your family member or yourself, developing a reliance on God or a higher power, and helping others in your own family or other families.

- *Reduce feelings of guilt and shame. Guilt* refers to feeling bad about what you did or didn't do (your behaviors). *Shame* refers to feeling bad about yourself and feeling like there is something wrong with you. Discuss these feelings with a counselor, religious leader, other concerned professional, or recovering family member. Don't blame yourself for your loved one's SUD. No one can change the past, but you can change the present and future. Use Al-Anon, Nar-Anon, or other family support programs to help you cope with guilt and shame.

- *Forgive your family member with the SUD.* This person probably did things to hurt, anger, embarrass, or shame you without intending to do so. Although she may have chosen to use alcohol or other drugs, she did not choose to develop an SUD. When you learn about SUDs and begin healing, you will be in better shape to let go of these feelings and work toward forgiving your family member. Don't be surprised if you struggle with this process. Give yourself time and don't judge yourself if it's hard to forgive. Forgiving is an act of love and courage. It will help you let go of anger and other feelings that have built up.

- *Forgive yourself.* You probably did some things yourself that hurt others as you got sucked into the grips of the SUD. You did the best you could under the circumstances. Remember, an SUD takes many victims. There is what a friend calls "collateral damage" to family members. The past is over and you cannot change it, but you can change how you view or feel about it. Be kind to yourself. If you are like most people, you are more forgiving to others than to yourself. You deserve self-compassion. You will also find it easier to forgive yourself if you make amends and undo damage that your behaviors caused with other family members.

- *Use your faith or your religion to gain strength.* Many of us have gained strength from our spiritual and religious practices. In mutual support programs, we are taught to rely on God or a power greater than ourselves to help change and deal with problems and struggles. Our faith has helped many of us get through difficult and painful times. Being grateful for what goes well, what you have in life, and for the chance to change can help, too. If you are an agnostic or atheist, use your connections with people you trust for help and support.

- *Share your experiences with other family members in recovery.* Once you have healed and changed, you may wish to share your experiences and strength with other suffering family members, both within your own family and in other families. The reason for the success of mutual support programs is that they enable people who have experienced a problem to help others in a similar situation. Don't rush into the role of helping before you've had a chance to receive help and support from others. Let others help you first, and take care of your own recovery before you worry about helping others. There is great joy and reward in giving back to others what was given to us.

MUTUAL SUPPORT PROGRAMS

These fellowships involve people with similar problems who help each other. Through sharing hope, experience, and strength, people support each other through the struggles and problems associated with SUDs and recovery. These programs help family members of loved ones with SUDs learn more about SUDs and recovery and how to engage in their own re-covery. Mutual support programs include:

- *Group meetings.* You listen to another member share his story of how he was affected by a loved one's SUD and how he learned not to let this dominate his life. You do not have to share your story at a meeting unless you want to and feel you have enough stable recovery under your belt. A sponsor in Al-Anon or Nar-Anon or other active member can help you figure out if you are ready to share. Some meetings discuss current concerns of members, or a topic such as relapse, serenity, or one of the 12 Steps or 12 Traditions. From these meetings, you learn information as well as new ideas on how to cope with your challenges in recovery. The most common mutual support programs for family members are Al-Anon, and Nar-Anon. There are also special support groups for parents. Do an internet search for programs in your area or consult your phone directory, local drug and alcohol clinics, or members of Al-Anon and Nar-Anon to find out about support groups available to you. Some treatment facilities offer family support groups.

- *Consider online meetings.* If you do not have easy access to meetings, check to see if online meetings are available. Many mutual support and other family programs offer online services. Some even offer access to family coaches or others to answer questions or guide you in recovery.

- *Sponsorship.* An experienced Al-Anon or Nar-Anon member takes a new member under her wing as she gets involved in the program. The sponsor serves as a sounding board, friend, and role model. She helps the new member use the tools of the programs such as the 12 Steps, recovery slogans, and literature.

- *The 12 Steps and slogans.* These are suggested steps to help you deal with your reactions to a loved one's SUD. They focus on you and help you change yourself. Slogans are sayings that help you coach yourself. Common ones are "one day at a time," "easy does it," "let go and let God," and "this too shall pass."

- *Literature and special events.* There are many pamphlets and books written for family members and friends. This literature can provide strategies that aid your recovery. Conventions and dinners offer the opportunity to get together with other family members in recovery on a social basis.

Every three years, Al-Anon conducts a survey of members. The most recent survey shows that 92% believe they were very positively affected by Al-Anon participation. Members endorse significant improvements in their mental health, physical health, work behaviors, and daily functioning.

RESOURCES ON THE WORLD WIDE WEB AND OTHER SOURCES

Recovery materials and websites provide you with information and coping ideas. These resources are written by recovering family members as well as professionals. Helpful resources include chatrooms in which you can join mutual support meetings with others. Chatrooms can be helpful when you don't have easy access to meetings in your community. Some resources offer the chance to speak to others on the phone to get information, support, and help finding treatment or recovery resources. The appendix near the end of this guide provides a list of resources with brief descriptions and contact information.

13

Helping Children Affected by a Parent's Substance Use Disorder

This chapter is for readers with children who have been affected by the SUD of a parent, sibling, or other family member. It is also for any reader interested in better understanding how SUDs impact children, and how these children can be helped by adults. In earlier chapters of this guide, we discussed that children of parents with SUDs are at increased risk for alcohol and drug use, behavior problems, school problems, depression and anxiety, and medical problems. Many studies, our clinical work with families, and personal experiences shared by children show that many are hurt by a parent's or sibling's SUD. This is true whether or not the child says anything or shows obvious signs of being affected. A child can appear fine on the outside but suffer quietly on the inside, especially if he keeps feelings, fears, and worries bottled up.

RESILIENCE

There are protective or offsetting factors—meaning that not all people, including children, are affected by a parent's SUD in the same way. Strong connections with school, religious community, adults and mentors (teachers, coaches, relatives, friends), and involvement in meaningful activities (academic, creative, athletic, social) may help offset some of the negative impact of living in a family with an SUD. Many children show resilience and cope with difficult situations, including having a parent with an SUD. Don't assume all children are affected the same way.

HOW CAN YOU HELP CHILDREN IMPACTED BY AN SUD IN THE FAMILY?

Here are different ways you can help your children if they were exposed to a family member's SUD.

Accept That Your Children Were Affected

Don't deny, minimize, or ignore the fact that children can be affected by SUDs. While you don't want to blame yourself for what the children have been through, accept that SUDs affect everyone in the family. Don't assume that your children weren't affected just because they don't say anything or show problems in school or other areas of life.

Talk with Your Children About Their Experiences

Encourage your children to talk about their experiences, feelings, worries, and concerns. Tell them that kids are often upset and have feelings about a family member with an SUD. Ask your children to share their feelings. Be gentle and supportive because it may take some prodding to get them to open up. Some kids who harbor upset feelings have trouble sharing these with others, even a parent or sibling who do not have SUD. If the family member with the SUD is sober and in a recovery program, encourage him to be part of these discussions.

Validate Your Children's Feelings

Whatever emotions are expressed to you, accept these as real for the child. Let your children know you can understand their feelings and want to hear what they have to say. Don't encourage the expression of feelings only to tell a child that she shouldn't feel a certain way. Don't be surprised to hear about anger, rage, anxiety, sadness, depression, loneliness, or confusion.

Be Available to Your Children

It isn't unusual for children to need to discuss feelings or experiences over and over. Give them the message that talking and asking for support from you is healthy and acceptable and that you are available to hear what they want to discuss. Encourage children to come to you to talk rather than letting feelings build up on the inside.

Educate Your Children

Children in a family with a member suffering from an SUD can develop incorrect beliefs about SUDs, the affected family member, or even themselves. For example, a child may think that alcohol is bad and not see that the problem isn't with alcohol but with a parent's alcohol use disorder. Or a child may think that he is responsible for the parent's drinking behaviors. Help the child understand that this person is sick, not bad. Provide education about substances, SUDs, treatment, and recovery so the children in the family have a better understanding.

If you discuss addiction as a medical disorder, explain that it has a hereditary component and often runs in families. Tell the child that addiction is considered a disease, and that scientists believe that there is something different in the brains of people with addiction compared to those who are not addicted. The webpage of the National Institute on Drug Abuse (www.nih.nida.gov) has many materials written for children to help them understand SUDs.

There are also many informative booklets, pamphlets, and books or brochures discussing SUDs, children of parents with SUDs, families, and other topics. Give readings to your children, and then discuss these readings with them.

Protect Your Children

Think safety first and do not tolerate violence. Seek immediate help from the police, a crisis intervention service, a shelter, a professional, or family and friends if any family member is violent or there has been any sexual abuse. If you tolerate abuse or violence, your children will feel unsafe and anxious. They may learn through observation that violence is acceptable and act out by getting into fights or physical altercations with others.

Promote Hope for Positive Change

If the family member with the SUD is not in treatment, let the children know that you are trying to get this member help. If the affected member is in treatment, tell the children that things won't be perfect, but they will get better in time. Let the children know that other family members' involvement in treatment will lead to things getting better in the family, too. Tell your children that treatment is where people with SUDs get help with their problems and learn how to live without alcohol or drugs. Also tell your children that community meetings (AA, NA, SMART Recovery, and others) help adults with alcohol or drug problems.

Share Activities

Spend time with the children, helping with homework and talking about school and friends. Do leisure or fun things together at home or outside of the home. Arrange special one-on-one time with each child so you can give him or her your sole attention.

Maintain Family Rituals

Respect the importance of family rituals such as having meals, watching television, doing yardwork, or engaging in tasks or activities together. Celebrate special occasions like birthdays, holidays, and graduations.

Show Interest in Your Children's Outside Activities

Attend school events with your children (sporting events, plays, concerts, and so on). Encourage the kids to focus not only on academics but on other activities as well, such as sports, music, arts and crafts, scouting, or social clubs at school.

Get Your Children Help If Needed

Problems that may require help include children acting out and getting in trouble in school (e.g., sassing teachers, skipping classes, poor grades), with friends (e.g., getting high or drunk with other kids, getting into fights, hanging with the wrong crowd), or in the community or with the law (e.g., underage drinking, stealing, setting fires).

Mental health problems include anxiety, depressive disorders, mood swings, talking about suicide or expressing a wish to be dead, attempting suicide, cutting or burning oneself, and hyperactivity (e.g., edginess, inability to sit still, troubling paying attention or concentrating on tasks at school or home). Ask the school counselor, your family doctor, or your religious leader for a recommendation on where to go for help. You can also call a local mental health clinic or look online or in the phone book under psychiatrists, psychologists, mental health specialists, or counselors and make an appointment. If you are in therapy yourself, ask your therapist or doctor for advice if you are concerned about any of your children.

Support Groups for Children

Some areas offer Alateen or other programs for children and teens of parents who have an SUD, but not enough of these programs exist. Check to see if they are available in your community. Get information about available programs and help your children understand how these support groups can help them as they begin to discuss their experiences with a parent's SUD.

You deserve a lot of credit for reading this guide. You have learned about:

- SUDs
- their impacts on you and your family
- recovery for your loved one with the SUD
- recovery for the family
- what you can do to help yourself

Although SUDs cause problems and heartache, they are highly treatable. Involvement in professional treatment and mutual support programs offers much hope to people with SUDs if they stick with these programs long enough.

Similarly, you as a family member affected by a loved one's SUD can grow as a person and feel better about yourself by getting involved in recovery. People from other families who have felt and experienced things similar to you can be a source of support and help. You do not have to go through this alone, and there are many things you can do to take more control over your life. We admire and applaud your efforts to help yourself and your family.

Helpful Resources

These resources provide a rich array of educational materials, recovery tools, and treatment and recovery resources for practitioners, individuals with substance-related disorders, and families or significant others who are affected by a loved one's substance problems. Many of these websites include free PDF files that you can save on your computer or print. For practitioners, many treatment manuals, research papers, and treatment protocols are available that address assessment and treatment of substance-related disorders. For individuals and families, many articles, guides, and information sheets on substances and treatment and recovery from substance-related problems are available. Some resources, such as many of the mutual support programs, include online meetings or chatrooms. Others provide phone numbers to call for information about treatment services, or for help and support for a family member or friend with an SUD or for yourself. You can also get information and referral information from local and state organizations that focus on helping individuals or families affected by substance-related problems. You may need to insert http:// before the website addresses.

US GOVERNMENT NATIONAL ORGANIZATIONS

1. **National Institute on Alcohol Abuse and Alcoholism (NIAAA)** provides information on alcohol, alcohol-related problems, treatment, and recovery. www.niaaa.nih.gov

2. **National Institute on Drug Abuse (NIDA)** provides information on all types of drugs, drug-related problems, treatment, and recovery. Includes information to help young kids and teens learn about how drugs affect the brain and behavior. www.nida.nih.gov

3. **Substance Abuse and Mental Health Services Administration (SAMHSA)** offers free, confidential help lines every day of the year, 24/7, to provide information, referral, and/or help for (a) individuals or families affected by an SUD or a mental health disorder (1-800-662-4357); (b) individuals in distress who are suicidal (1-800-273-8255); and (c) individuals in distress who need crisis help due to a disaster (1-800-985-5990). www.samhsa.gov

MUTUAL SUPPORT PROGRAMS FOR ALCOHOL OR DRUG PROBLEMS

1. **Alcoholics Anonymous (AA)** is a mutual support program for anyone with an alcohol problem who wants to stop drinking. AA has tools such as recovery meetings, sponsorship, recovery literature, the 12-step program, and many other resources. www.aa.org. AA online chat meetings are also available at www.aa-alive.net.

2. **Alcoholics Victorious** is a program for individuals with alcohol or drug problems that uses the 12 steps of AA and readings from the Bible to promote recovery, with a focus on using Jesus as the higher power. www.alcoholicsvictorious.org

3. **Narcotics Anonymous (NA)** is a mutual support program for individuals with any type of drug problem. It offers tools such as recovery meetings, sponsorship, recovery literature, the 12-step program, and other resources. www.na.org. NA Online Chat meetings are also available at www.nachatroom.org.

4. **SMART Recovery (Self-Management and Recovery Training)** is a program for recovery from all types of addiction, including alcohol and drug addictions. It offers a four-point program, meetings in person or online, chatrooms, and recovery literature. www.smartrecovery.org

5. **Women for Sobriety** is a program that helps women find their individual path to recovery through discovery of self, gained by sharing experiences, hopes, and encouragement with other women in similar circumstances. Online meetings are available as well as a meeting finder. womenforsobriety.org/about

FAMILY RESOURCES

1. **Al-Anon** is a mutual support program for friends and families of individuals with alcohol problems. Al-Anon offers group meetings (in person, by phone, online, international) where friends and family members share their experiences and learn ways to cope with the effects of the alcohol problem on themselves. al-anon.org. Al-Anon online chat meetings are available on www.stepchat.com/alanon.htm.

2. **Alateen** is a program for teens whose lives have been affected by someone else's drinking. Like Al-Anon, Alateen provides group meetings where members share experiences and learn the principles of the Al-Anon program. al-anon.org/newcomers/teen-corner-alateen

3. **Community Reinforcement Approach and Family Training (CRAFT)** is an approach to help families and significant others deal with a substance use problem in the family. It provides guidance on how to engage the member with the substance problem in treatment. It also helps the family deal with their own reactions to a loved one and to engage in their own recovery. www.robertjmeyersphd.com/craft

4. **Dr. Dennis C. Daley's website** includes treatment manuals for professionals and recovery materials for individuals and family members covering SUDs, psychiatric disorders, and co-occurring disorders (both disorders combined). www. drdenniscdaley.com

5. **Faces and Voices of Recovery** is an advocacy organization that provides information and support for families and those with an SUD. www.facesandvoicesofrecovery.org

6. **Facing Addiction** is an advocacy organization dedicated to finding solutions to the addiction crisis. They aim to build a national constituency, increase access to treatment, translate scientific innovation into services, advocate for governments to implement evidence-based policies, and share the proof of long-term recovery. www.facingaddiction.org

7. **Family Resource Center** offers various resources for families to understand and address a child's substance use. The resources can be filtered by the intended user—for example, parents of young adolescents, older teens, adult children, or teachers/ community support personnel. www.familyresourcectr.org/ category/community

8. **Families Anonymous** is for the families and friends who have known a feeling of desperation concerning the destructive behavior of someone very near to them, whether caused by drugs, alcohol, or related behavioral problems. Meetings without Walls are online meetings. www.familiesanonymous.org

9. **Nar-Anon** is a 12-step mutual support program adopted from NA. This program offers group meetings and recovery tools for families affected by any type of drug problem. www.nar-anon.org/

10. **National Association of Children of Alcoholics** offers a rich array of information and resources on substance use problems and recovery for families and children of all ages, and for professionals. You can access written and video materials, webinars, research reports, and stories of recovery of family members affected by a loved one's SUD. www.nacoa.org

11. **Partnership for Drug-Free Kids** is a nonprofit organization that aims to help families struggling with their son or daughter's substance use. They provide information, support, and guidance to families, in addition to advocating for greater understanding and more effective programs to treat addiction. They offer a helpline that helps families connect with experts. www.drugfree.org

12. **SAMSHA—20-Minute Guide** is a free online resource for parents and partners about how they can help change their children's substance use. https://the20minuteguide.com

REFERENCES AND SUGGESTED READINGS

Ackerman, R. (1987). *Children of alcoholics: A guide for parents, educators, and therapists* (2nd ed.). New York, NY: Simon & Schuster.

Ackerman, R. (2002). *Perfect daughters: Adult daughters of alcoholics* (2nd ed.). Hollywood, FL: HCI.

Al-Anon Family Group. (1981). *Alateen: Hope for children of alcoholics*. New York, NY: Al-Anon Family Group Headquarters, Inc.

Al-Anon Family Group. (1984). *Al-Anon faces alcoholism* (2nd ed.). New York, NY: Al-Anon Family Group Headquarters, Inc.

Al-Anon Family Group. (2016). *2015 membership survey: Results and longitudinal comparison*. Retrieved from www.Al-Anon.org.

American Psychiatric Association. (2013). Substance-related disorders. In *Diagnostic and statistical manual of mental disorders* (5th ed.). Washington, DC: American Psychiatric Association.

American Society of Addiction Medicine. (2015). *Principles of addiction medicine* (5th ed.). Chevy Chase, MD: American Society of Addiction Medicine.

Andreas-Burdzovic, J., & O'Farrell, T. (2007). Longitudinal associations between fathers' heavy drinking patterns and children's psychosocial adjustment. *Journal of Abnormal Child Psychology, 35*, 1–16.

Center for Substance Abuse Treatment. (2000). *Substance abuse treatment reduces family dysfunction, improves productivity*. Rockville, MD: Center for Substance Abuse Treatment.

Conners, N. A., Bradley, R. H., Mansell, L. W., Liu, J. Y., Roberts, T. J., Burgdorf, K., & Herrell, J. (2004). Children of mothers with serious substance abuse problems: An accumulation of risks. *American Journal of Drug and Alcohol Abuse, 30*(1), 85–100.

Cooke, C. G., Kelley, M., Fals-Stewart, W., & Golden, J. (2005). A comparison of the psychosocial functioning of children with drug-versus alcohol-dependent fathers. *American Journal of Drug and Alcohol Abuse, 30*(4), 695–710.

Cork, M. (1969). *The forgotten children*. Toronto, Canada: Alcoholism and Drug Addiction Research Foundation.

Daley, D. (2017). Grief has no expiration date. Part 1: Losing a loved one to addiction. *Counselor, 18*(4), 19–22.

Daley, D. (2017). Grief has no expiration date. Part 2: Coping with the loss of a loved one to addiction. *Counselor, 18*(5), 24–26.

Daley, D., & Douaihy A. (2010). *A family guide to addiction and recovery.* Murrysville, PA: Daley Publications.

Daley, D., & Douaihy, A. (2013). Co-occurring disorders. In A. Douaihy & D. Daley (Eds.), *Substance use disorders: Pittsburgh pocket psychiatry* (pp. 283–310). New York, NY: Oxford University Press.

Daley, D., & Douaihy, A. (2015). *Relapse prevention counseling: Clinical strategies to guide addiction recovery and reduce relapse.* Eau Claire, WI: PESI Publishing & Media, Inc.

Daley, D., & Douaihy, A. (2017). Drug use disorders. In A. Wenzel (Ed.), *The SAGE encyclopedia of abnormal and clinical psychology* (pp. 1196–1200). Thousand Oaks, CA: SAGE Publications, Inc.

Daley, D., & Tartar, R. (2017). Children of parents with substance use disorder. In A. Wenzel (Ed.), *The SAGE encyclopedia of abnormal and clinical psychology* (pp. 643–644). Thousand Oaks, CA: SAGE Publications, Inc.

Daley, D. C. (2003). *Understanding suicide and addiction.* Center City, MN: Hazelden.

Daley, D. C. (2013). *Relapse prevention workbook.* Export, PA: Daley Publications.

Daley, D. C., & Miller, J. (2001). *Addiction in your family.* Holmes Beach, FL: Learning Publications.

Daley, D. C., & Moss, H. M. (2002). *Dual disorders: Counseling clients with chemical dependency and mental illness* (3rd ed.). Center City, MN: Hazelden.

Daley, D. C., & Spear, J. (2003). *A family guide to coping with dual disorders* (2nd ed.). Center City, MN: Hazelden.

Douaihy, A., & Daley, D. (2013). *Substance use disorders: Pittsburgh pocket psychiatry.* New York, NY: Oxford University Press.

Gaines, W. S. (2011). *Blood on a pew.* Mustang, OK: Tate Publishing Co.

Jansson, L., & Velez, M. (2010). Neonatal abstinence syndrome. *Current Opinion in Pediatrics, 24*(2), 252–258.

Jones, H., Kaltenbach, K., Heil, S. H., Stine, S. M., Coyle, M. G., Arria, A. M., . . . Fischer, G. (2010). Neonatal abstinence syndrome after methadone or buprenorphine exposure. *New England Journal of Medicine, 363*(24), 2320–2332.

Kaufman, E., & Yoshioka, M. (2004). *Substance abuse and family therapy. Treatment improvement protocol, TIP39.* Rockville, MD: Substance Abuse and Mental Health Services Administration.

Kelly, J. F. (2016). *The science on the effectiveness and mechanisms of AA and 12-step treatments.* ATTC SAMHSA webinar, April 21, 2016.

Kelly, J. F., Bergman, B., Hoeppner, B. B., Vilsaint, C., & White, W. L. (2017). Prevalence, pathways, and predictors of recovery from drug and alcohol problems in the United States population: Implications for practice, research, and policy. *Drug and Alcohol Dependence, 181*, 162–169.

Kelly, T., & Daley, D. (2013). Integrated treatment of substance use and psychiatric disorders. *Social Work in Public Health, 28*(3-4), 388–406.

Kendler, K. S., Ohlsson, H., Sundquist, J., & Sundquist, K. (2016). Alcohol use disorder and mortality across the lifespan: A longitudinal cohort and co-relative analysis. *Journal of the American Medical Association, 73*(6), 575–581.

Kessler, R., Crum, R. M., Warner, L. A., Nelson, C. B., Schulenberg, J., & Anthony, J. C. (1997). Lifetime co-occurrence of DSM-III-R alcohol abuse and dependence with other psychiatric disorders in the National Comorbidity Survey. *Archives of General Psychiatry, 54*, 313–321.

Kirisci, L., Vanyukov, M., & Tarter, R. (2005). Detection of youth at high risk for substance use disorders: A longitudinal study. *Psychology of Addictive Behaviors, 19*(3), 243–252.

Klostermann, K., & O'Farrell, T. (2013). Treating substance abuse: Partner and family approaches. *Social Work in Public Health, 28*(3-4), 234–247.

Kmiec, J., Cornelius, J., & Douaihy, A. (2013). Pharmacotherapy of substance use disorders. In A. Douaihy & D. Daley (Eds.), *Substance use disorders: Pittsburgh pocket psychiatry* (pp. 169–212). New York, NY: Oxford University Press.

Kraft, W. K., Adeniyi-Jones, S. C., Chervoneva, I., Greenspan, J. S., Abatemarco, D., Kaltenbach, K., & Ehrlich, M.E. (2017). Buprenorphine for the treatment of the neonatal abstinence syndrome. *New England Journal of Medicine, 376*, 2341–2348.

Landau, J., Garrett, J., Shea, R. R., Stanton, M. D., Brinkman-Sull, D., & Baciewicz, G. (2000). Strength in numbers: The ARISE method for mobilizing family and network to engage substance abusers in treatment. *American Journal of Drug and Alcohol Abuse, 26*(3), 379–398.

Lander, L., Howsare, J., & Byrne, M. (2013). The impact of substance use disorders on families and children. *Social Work in Public Health, 28*(3–4), 194–203.

Laudet, A. (2013). *Life in recovery: Report on the survey findings.* Washington, DC: Faces and Voices of Recovery.

Liddle, H. A., Dakof, G. A., Parker, K., Diamond, G. S., Barrett, K., & Tejeda, M. (2001). Multidimensional family therapy for adolescent drug abuse: Results of a randomized clinical trial. *American Journal of Drug and Alcohol Abuse, 27*(4), 651–688.

Liepman, M. R., Gross, K. A., Lagos, M. E., Parran Jr., T. V., & Farkas, K. J. (2014). Family involvement in addiction, treatment and recovery. In R. K. Ries, D. A. Fiellin, S. C. Miller, & R. Saitz (Eds.), *The ASAM principles of addiction medicine* (5th ed., pp. 958–974). New York, NY: Wolters Kluwer.

Marlatt, A., & Donovan, D. (2004). *Relapse prevention* (2nd ed.) New York, NY: Guilford Press.

McLellan, A. T., Lewis, D. C., O'Brien, C. P., & Kleber, H. D. (2000). Drug dependence, a chronic medical illness: Implications for treatment, insurance, and outcome evaluation. *Journal of the American Medical Association, 284*(13), 1689–1695.

Meyers, R., Miller, W. R., Hill, D. E., & Tonigan, J. S. (1999). Community Reinforcement and Family Training (CRAFT): Engaging unmotivated drug users in treatment. *Journal of Substance Abuse, 10*(3), 291–308.

Meyers, R. H., & Wolfe, B. L. (2004). *Getting your loved one sober: Alternatives to nagging, pleading and threatening.* Center City, MN: Hazelden.

Miller, W. R., & Rollnick, S. (2015). *Motivational interviewing: Preparing people to change addictive behavior* (3rd ed.). New York, NY: Guilford Press.

Minear, S., & Zuckerman, B. (2013). Interventions for children of substance-using parents. In N. Suchman, M. Pajulo, & L. Mayes (Eds.), *Parenting and substance abuse: Developmental approaches to intervention* (pp. 235–257). New York, NY: Oxford University Press.

Moe, J. (2007). *Understanding addiction and recovery through a child's eyes: Hope, help, and healing for families.* Deerfield Beach, FL: Health Communications, Inc.

Moss, H., Vanyukov, M., Majumder, P. P., Kirisci, L., & Tarter, R. E. (1995). Prepubertal sons of substance abusers: Influences of paternal and familial substance abuse on behavioral disposition, IQ and school achievement. *Addictive Behaviors, 20,* 1–14.

Mueser, K. T., Noordsy, D. L., Drake, R. E., & Fox, L. (2003). *Integrated treatment for dual disorders: A guide for effective practice.* New York, NY: Guildford Press.

National Academies of Science, Engineering, Medicine. (2017). *The health effects of cannabis and cannabinoids: Current state of evidence and recommendations.* Washington, DC: National Academies Press.

National Center on Addiction and Substance Abuse at Columbia University. (2012). *Addiction medicine: Closing the gap between science and practice.* New York, NY: National Center on Addiction and Substance Abuse at Columbia University.

National Institute on Alcohol Abuse and Alcoholism (NIAAA). (2017). *Fetal alcohol exposure.* Retrieved from http://www.niaaa.nih.gov/alcohol-health/fetal-alcohol-exposure.

National Institute on Drug Abuse. (2012). *Principles of drug addiction treatment: A research-based guide* (3rd ed.). NIH Pub No. 12-4180. Bethesda, MD: US Department of Health and Human Services.

Nunes, E. V., Selzer, J., Levounis, P., & Davies, C. A. (2010). *Substance dependence and co-occurring psychiatric disorders: Best practices for diagnosis and clinical treatment.* Kingston, NJ: Civic Research Institute.

Nunes, E. V., Weissman, M. M., Goldstein, R., McAvay, G., Beckford, C., Seracini, A., . . . Wickramaratne, P. (2000). Psychiatric disorders and impairment in the children of opiate addicts: Prevalences and distribution by ethnicity. *American Journal on Addictions, 9,* 232–241.

Orford, J., Velleman, R., Natera, G., Templeton, L., & Copello, A. (2013). Addiction in the family is a major but neglected contributor to the global burden of adult ill-health. *Elsevier Social Science & Medicine, 78,* 70–77.

Regier, D. (1990). Comorbidity of mental disorders with alcohol and other drug abuse: Results from the epidemiologic catchment area study. *Journal of the American Medical Association, 264,* 2511–2518.

Rowe, C. L. (2012). Family therapy for drug abuse: Review and updates 2003–2010. *Journal of Marital & Family Therapy, 38*(1), 59–81.

Schwartzmier, M. (2017). *My daughter died from an overdose. I'm sharing her story to help others.* Partnership for Drug-Free Kids. Retrieved from https://drugfree.org/parent-blog/my-daughter-died-from-an-overdose-im-sharing-her-story-to-help-others/.

Smith, E., & Daley, D. (2017). Substance use disorders and the family. In A. Wenzel (Ed.), *The SAGE encyclopedia of abnormal and clinical psychology* (pp. 3378–3882). Thousand Oaks, CA: SAGE Publications.

Smith, J., & Meyers, R. (2004). *Motivating substance abusers to enter treatment: Working with family members. The CRAFT intervention program.* New York, NY: Guilford Press.

Solis, J., Shadur, J. M., Burns, A. R., & Hussong, A. M. (2012). Understanding the diverse needs of children whose parents abuse substances. *Current Drug Abuse Reviews*, *5*(2), 135–137.

Stanton, M. D., & Shadish, W. R. (1997). Outcome, attrition, and family-couples treatment for drug abuse: A meta-analysis and review of the controlled, comparative studies. *Psychological Bulletin*, *122*(2), 170–191.

Substance Abuse and Mental Health Services Administration. (2009). *National registry of evidence-based programs and practices (NREPP)*. Retrieved from www.nrepp.samhsa.gov.

Substance Abuse and Mental Health Services Administration. (2013). *Addressing fetal alcohol spectrum disorders (FASD). Treatment improvement protocol, TIP58*. DHHS Publication No. (SMA) 13-4803. Rockville, MD: Substance Abuse and Mental Health Services Administration.

Substance Abuse and Mental Health Services Administration. (2015). *Medication for the treatment of alcohol use disorders*. DHSS Publication No. (SMA) 15-4907. Rockville, MD: Substance Abuse and Mental Health Services Administration

Substance Abuse and Mental Health Services Administration. (2015). *Medication-assisted treatment of opioid use disorder*. DHSS Publication No. (SMA) 14-4892R. Rockville, MD: Substance Abuse and Mental Health Services Administration.

Substance Abuse and Mental Health Services Administration. (2016). *Building systems together for family recovery, safety and stability*. Webinar sponsored by SAMHSA and the Administration for Children and Families Children's Bureau, September 6, 2017.

Substance Abuse and Mental Health Services Administration. (2016). *A collaborative approach to the treatment of pregnant women with opioid use disorder*. DHHS Publication No. (SMA) 16–4978. Rockville, MD: Substance Abuse and Mental Health Services Administration.

Substance Abuse and Mental Health Services Administration. (2017). *2016 survey on drug use and health*. Rockville, MD: Substance Abuse and Mental Health Services Administration.

Suchman, N., Pajulo, M., & Mayes, L. (2013). *Parenting and substance abuse: Developmental approaches to intervention*. New York, NY: Oxford University Press.

Szapocznik, J., Hervis, O., & Schwartz, S. (2003). *Brief strategic family therapy for adolescent drug abuse*. Bethesda, MD: National Institute on Drug Abuse.

Tarter, R., Blackson, T., Brigham, J., Moss, H., & Caprara, G. V. (1995). The association between childhood irritability and liability to substance use in early adolescence: A two-year follow-up study of boys at risk for substance abuse. *Drug and Alcohol Dependence*, *39*, 253–261.

US Department of Health and Human Services. (2016). *Facing addiction in America: The Surgeon General's report on alcohol, drugs and health*. Rockville, MD: US Department of Health and Human Services.

Viteri, O., Soto, E. E., Bahado-Singh, R. O., Christensen, C. W., Chauhan, S. P., & Sibai, B. M. (2015). Fetal anomalies and long-term effects associated with substance abuse in pregnancy: A literature review. *American Journal of Perinatology*, *32*(5), 405–416.

Volkow, N. D., & Collins, F. (2017). The role of science in addressing the opioid crisis. *New England Journal of Medicine*, *377*, 391–394.

Volkow, N. D., Compton, W. M., & Weiss, S. R. (2014). Adverse health effects of marijuana use. *New England Journal of Medicine, 23*, 2219–2227.

Volkow, N. D., & Fowler, J. S. (2000). Addiction, a disease of compulsion and
drive: Involvement of the orbitofrontal cortex. *Cerebral Cortex, 10*, 318–325.

Wallace, K. (2014). *Being an addict's mom: It's just a very, very sad place.* Retrieved
August 24, 2014, from www.cnn.com.

Ward, J., & Daley, D. (2014). A parent's journey to recovery. *Counselor Connection,
8*(Dec), 4.

White, W. L. (2017). *Groundbreaking survey of recovery pathways.* Retrieved from www.
williamwhitepapers.

White, W. L. (2017). *Recovery rising.* Lexington, KY: Rita Chaney, Publisher.

White, W. L., & Daley, D. (2016). *Calling attention to opioid-affected families and children.* Retrieved from www.williamwhitepapers.com.

Wolin, S. J., & Wolin, S. (1993). *The resilient self: How survivors of troubled families rise
above adversity.* New York, NY: Villard Guides.

Dennis C. Daley, PhD, is Senior Clinical Director of Substance Use Services in the Behavioral Health Integration Division at the University of Pittsburgh Medical Center Insurance Division. He is also a professor of psychiatry at the University of Pittsburgh School of Medicine. Dr. Daley has been involved in clinical care, research, and teaching about addiction for nearly 40 years. He has conducted hundreds of presentations in the United States, Canada, Europe, Mexico, Taiwan, and Vietnam.

Dr. Daley previously served for 14 years as Chief of Addiction Medicine Services at Western Psychiatric Institute and Clinic (WPIC) and 11 years as the Director and Principal Investigator of the Appalachian Tri-State Node of the National Institute on Drug Abuse's Clinical Trials Network, housed at WPIC. He has been an investigator, consultant, and trainer on numerous local and national studies.

He published the first book in the United States for counselors, and the first recovery workbooks for individuals and families on substance use disorders and co-occurring psychiatric disorders. He was also one of the first in the United States to publish interactive workbooks on recovery from addiction. For decades, Dr. Daley has advocated for recovery for individuals and families affected by addiction.

Dr. Daley served on the Veterans Administration's MIRECC Project for over 12 years in consulting and educational capacities related to addition and mental health services for veterans. He has been involved in several national and local organizations that address substance use issues.

Dr. Daley has over 400 publications, including books, chapters, articles, and recovery guides. He writes regular columns for *Counselor* and other publications. He created over 35 educational videos on recovery from addiction, mental health disorders, or co-occurring disorders, including the *Living Sober* series for addiction and the *Promise of Recovery* series for mental health disorders. His treatment manuals and his patient or family recovery materials are used in many programs in the United States and other countries. Several of his writings have been translated into foreign languages. He has also published material for children on understanding substance use problems.

Antoine Douaihy, MD, is professor of psychiatry and medicine at the University of Pittsburgh School of Medicine. He also serves as the senior academic director of Addiction Medicine Services and director of the Addiction Psychiatry Fellowship at Western Psychiatric Hospital of the University of Pittsburgh Medical Center. He has a well-established career in patient care/advocacy, education, training, and research in the areas of motivational interviewing, substance use disorders, co-occurring disorders, and HIV/AIDS. He and Dr. Daley have worked together for 20 years providing clinical services, conducting clinical research, teaching and mentoring healthcare practitioners and medical trainees, and publishing. In recognition for his dedication to an academic career, Dr. Douaihy has been the recipient of multiple awards, including the Leonard Tow Humanism in Medicine Award and the Charles Watson Teaching Award, recognizing him for the qualities of a masterful clinician, academician, caretaker of his patients, educator, mentor, and contributor to the medical school community and the community at large.

For the benefit of digital users, indexed terms that span two pages (e.g., 52–53) may, on occasion, appear on only one of those pages.